BOOK THREE

INJURY, DISEASE & NURSING

Essential Equine Studies

BOOK THREE

INJURY, DISEASE & NURSING

JULIE BREGA

J. A. Allen
LONDON

ACKNOWLEDGEMENTS

Thanks to:

Sincere thanks to the many professional friends and colleagues for their invaluable contributions, advice and support over the years; without them The Open College could not have developed and progressed with such success.

Special thanks to my husband Bill and my daughter, Zoe for their support, hard work and enthusiasm for all of our projects.

Dedicated with love to Holly, Josh and George.

© *Julie Brega, 2007*
First published in Great Britain 2007

ISBN 978 0 85131 915 5
J.A. Allen
Clerkenwell House
Clerkenwell Green
London EC1R 0HT

J.A. Allen is an imprint of Robert Hale Limited

The right of Julie Brega to be identified as author
of this work has been asserted by her in accordance
with the Copyright, Designs and Patents Act 1988

A catalogue record for this book is available from the British Library

Design by Judy Linard
Edited by Martin Diggle
Illustrations by the author, except for the photograph on page 50
reproduced by kind permission of ECB Equine Ltd.,
and the photographs on pages 122–6 reproduced by kind permission
of Rossdale's Equine Hospital

Printed by New Era Printing Co. Limited, China

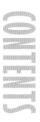

CONTENTS

LIST OF FIGURES

LIST OF TABLES

CHAPTER I
ACCIDENT PREVENTION AND EQUINE FIRST AID

The aims and objectives of this chapter are to explain:

- How to reduce the risk of accidents occurring.
- Which items are needed in the equine first aid kit.
- What constitutes an 'emergency'.

Knowledge of equine first aid is essential for anyone with responsibility for horses. Whether horses are kept for leisure, commercial or competitive use, there is always the chance that an accident will happen, resulting in injury. The information given in this chapter does not attempt to replace veterinary expertise; it should, however, enable you to liaise with the veterinary surgeon in an effective way.

You should also take into account the constant advancement of veterinary technology and the knowledge and understanding of disease in the horse. This is where reference to equestrian journals and magazines can be beneficial – they cover most new products on the market and publish information about new developments in veterinary medicine. Also, when possible, attend lectures and seminars to obtain new information.

Injuries arise as a result of all sorts of accidents – some horses even manage to injure themselves without setting foot out of the stable. In the first section of this chapter we will look at ways of reducing the chances of an accident occurring. However, even with the best care in the world, horses do get injured and it is important to recognize an emergency and deal with it promptly. Knowing what to do whilst waiting for the vet can make the difference between life and death (or permanent disablement).

ACCIDENT PREVENTION

As the saying goes, 'Prevention is better than cure'. Before we discuss first aid, wounds, healing, etc., it is good idea to think about how to prevent accidents from happening in the first place. While we can look at accident prevention in a number of distinct situations, we should realize that the underlying criteria of due care and common sense apply in all circumstances.

HANDLER TRAINING

- Many accidents are caused through lack of skill and experience on the part of the handler. Anyone working with horses, or even simply handling them, should receive thorough training in all aspects of their management. This should involve safety and accident prevention measures.

- Inexperienced handlers should work under close supervision and under the guidance of an experienced person. The inexperienced handler must not work with difficult or very young horses.

IN THE YARD AND STABLE

- Keep the yard tidy, free from debris, tools, equipment and haynets, which could injure a horse or trip someone over.

- Do not allow empty haynets to hang low in the stable. The horse may get a foot entangled.

- Keep the yard gate closed at all times – then at least if a horse breaks loose, he is contained.

- To prevent stabled horses from escaping, make sure top and bottom bolts on doors are securely bolted, especially last thing at night: use secure 'horse-proof' bolts.

- Keep the feed room door securely closed. If an escaped horse gorges himself in the feed room it could result in colic.

- Do not leave a horse loose in a stable wearing a nylon headcollar. The headcollar can become caught on the top bolt of the stable door, causing the horse to pull back and panic. A nylon headcollar may not break and the horse could be injured.

- Stables should be solidly constructed. Flimsy materials will splinter or break if the horse kicks out whilst rolling, etc. Make sure that stables are free from sharp projections such as nails.

- Stables should be well bedded down to prevent the horse from slipping. Sides that are banked up well can help to prevent the horse from becoming cast. Horses can damage themselves thrashing about when they become cast. Anti-cast strips can be fitted on the stable walls to give the horse's hind legs something to push against if he finds himself stuck on his back.

- Rubber matting generally provides non-slip flooring – although some types are slippery when wet. Add a small amount of bedding, e.g. shavings, to absorb urine and prevent the matting from getting too wet.

- Windows should be glazed with clear plastic or safety glass, which is then protected by a metal grille to prevent the horse injuring himself.

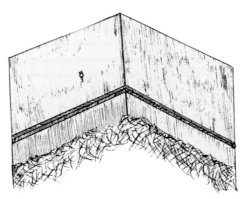

Figure 1 Anti-cast strips

TYING UP

- Only tie horses to tying rings securely fitted to a solid object, e.g. the wall. The tying ring should never be fixed onto something which may pull away, e.g. a loose rail or similar.

- Attach a weak link to the tying ring. This can be a loop of baler twine or string. Always tie the horse to the weak link so that, in the event that he pulls backwards, the weak link will break, rather than the headcollar. Use a quick-release knot so you can undo the rope in an emergency.

- Never leave horses tied up close to each other, as they may fight.

- Tie up so that the rope is not so long that the horse can put a foot over it and not so short that the horse becomes upset.

- Never tie up by the reins. The horse will injure his mouth or break the bridle if he pulls back.

- Never leave a horse unattended when tied up.

- When a young horse is tied up, e.g. for the farrier, have an assistant who can hold the horse if necessary. If the horse continually pulls back and breaks free, the farrier may be tempted to tie the horse directly to the tying ring, with potentially disastrous results. You have a responsibility to assist the farrier – this is for his benefit as well as your horse's.

IN THE FIELD

- *Never* use barbed wire as fencing for horses. Very serious injuries are caused when horses become entangled in barbed wire.

- If plain wire fencing is used, a wooden top rail must be used to help the horses see the fence when galloping around. It also stops them from leaning on the fence and causing the wire to sag.

- Never use pig netting as fencing for horses – the gaps are large enough for a horse to put a foot through. Once entangled, serious injuries can result as the horse panics to free himself.

- The fencing should be high enough to deter the horses from jumping out. The top rail should be at least 1.2 m (4 ft) high. The bottom rail should be high enough to stop a horse putting a foot over it but not so high that a pony or foal could roll underneath it.

- Check all fencing materials for safety – broken rails need to be repaired promptly and protruding nails removed. Check that no rails protrude into the field, e.g. slip rails must be fully opened before leading horses through. Slip rails must never be left partially closed when horses are loose in adjoining fields: serious injuries can result if the horses canter past protruding rails.

- Serious injuries can be caused by horses getting a foot caught in the gate. Ideally, gates should have vertical bars or a close wire mesh base. Metal five-bar gates are particularly dangerous as the horse can get a foot trapped in the V-shaped sections between the bars.

- Horses are particularly prone to injuries when they are in separate but adjoining fields as they may fight over the fence. This is when they are most likely to put a foot through the fence or gate, or try to kick each other. Ideally, there should be a gap between fence lines wide enough to drive a tractor and grass cutter through. If this is not possible, use a strip of electric fencing along the top of the rails to keep the horses away from the fence.

- Never leave a horse out in the field wearing a nylon headcollar. If the headcollar becomes caught up, it may not break and could cause serious injury.

- In confined paddocks, turn horses known to get on with each other out in small groups. The smaller the group, the less likely they are to fight. This is not such a problem in large paddocks. The more space the horses have, the less likely they are to fight.

- Introduce new members to the group carefully. Let the horses meet in the yard before turning them out together. Watch them and remove one if they do not get on.

- When turning a horse out for the first time, e.g. after box rest or similar, use the smallest paddock available to prevent him from galloping around too energetically. A round pen is ideal. Seek the vet's advice about the need to sedate the horse to prevent him injuring himself. Put brushing and overreach boots on if the horse is likely to charge around at first.

- Make sure the water trough doesn't have any sharp protrusions.

- Trim back sharp branches on hedges and trees.

- Fill in rabbit holes as a horse can be injured if he puts a foot down one whilst cantering around the field.

- Each horse's feet should be picked out at least twice a day and his legs checked for small cuts and wounds. A puncture wound can be hard to see and yet it can lead to an infection and time off work. Puncture wounds to the foot can be very serious, as the navicular bursa may be damaged. The earlier these are detected, the better.

ITQ 1 Give two examples of accidents that can happen whilst the horse is turned out in the field.

1.

2.

WHEN RIDDEN

- Brushing boots all round provide protection for flatwork and jumping. Overreach boots prevent tread injuries on the heels when jumping, and knee boots offer protection in the event of slipping on a hard surface, such as a worn/wet road.

- Keep horses out of kicking reach of each other, particularly if one is known to kick. In company, e.g. at a show, a kicker should wear a red ribbon in his tail to act as a warning to other riders.

- Tack and equipment must be safe and fit well. Accidents to both horse and rider can be caused by unsafe tack.

- Make sure the horse is fit enough to perform the task required. For example, if competing in horse trials, the horse must be fit enough to gallop around the cross-country course and jump the obstacles without undue stress. If not fit enough, the horse will be likely to tire quickly, possibly resulting in hitting a fence and/or falling. Tendon injuries are also more likely when the horse is not fit enough. The muscles tire earlier, resulting in the tendons taking extra strain.

- Wherever possible, work the horse on a safe, non-slip surface. This is not always possible so common sense must prevail. It would be foolish to lunge or jump (or, indeed, do any form of riding) on icy ground. Young horses in particular lack balance in the early stages of training and need to work on secure footing.

BASIC SAFETY WHEN RIDING ON THE ROAD

- Horses should always wear protective boots, including knee boots, when out hacking, and road studs can be fitted to the shoes of horses who work regularly on the roads to provide extra grip.

- Hack young or traffic-shy horses out with a sensible companion to set them a good example and instil confidence.

- If hacking out in a group, everyone must remember that they have to obey the rules of the road like any other road user. Stay on the left-hand side. If the road width permits, riders can go two abreast, but they should know how to resume single file quickly again if necessary.

- The leading escort should make constant checks of the ride and should always be aware of the traffic in front and to the rear.

- Riders should never allow gaps to develop into which vehicles could slot and thus divide the group up. The group should be maintained as a single unit, so when one horse turns across the road, all of the ride follows in close order.

- It is always a good idea to wear reflective jackets or arm-bands when hacking in case you get caught out by failing light, fog or generally murky conditions. The horses can wear leg-bands made of similar material. Stirrup lights, which shine white to the front and red to the back can also be fitted. However, if visibility is poor, or likely to become so, it is safer to avoid going on the roads.

- It is also safer to avoid busy roads, built-up areas and known hazards such as working heavy plant, which can spook horses. However, in the modern countryside, this is less and less easy to do.

- Courtesy to all pedestrians and road users should become second nature, to ensure that they return the compliment next time they pass a rider on the road. A smile and a nod cost nothing, but pay dividends when you meet them on the road again.

TRAVELLING

- The horse should always wear protective gear when travelling in a lorry or trailer. This includes leg bandages or travel boots, tail bandage and tail guard, and a poll guard. Knee and hock boots could also be fitted but bear in mind that not all horses will tolerate hock boots.

- The vehicle used for transporting the horses should be safe. This applies in particular to trailers. The floor should be solid and secure – if wooden it must not be worn or rotten. There have been horror stories of horses who have put a foot through the floor unbeknown to the driver, who carried on to complete the journey.

- The ramp must not be too steep, and should be very solid and non-slip. Secure rubber matting or rubber compound (as used on the main floor of many vehicles) and wooden slats provide a good purchase for the horse and prevent slipping. Wooden ramps, especially those with bits of old carpet nailed onto them, are not safe. Metal ramps are also slippery and make a loud noise as the horse walks on them.

- The ramp should have safe guides on each side to help keep the horse on it. Injuries are common after horses slip off the ramp, which may happen to horses who are young or misbehaving.

- The floor of the lorry or trailer must be non-slip. Rubber matting or a rubber compound is ideal. The latter is a rubber granule mixture which is laid on the floor and sets to form a solid, non-slip surface.

- Travel the horse with sufficient space to keep his balance. Horses need to spread their legs slightly apart to keep balanced. If the space is too small and restrictive, it can make the horse panic, possibly resulting in a fall.

- There must be no sharp projections, catches, etc. upon which the horse or his rugs can be snagged.

- Drive with consideration. Brake and accelerate gradually to allow horses time to adjust their balance. Take it steady round corners. A good adage to follow is, 'Drive as though you have a bucket of water in the boot and do not want to spill any.'

IN-TEXT ACTIVITY

Think of one or two examples of accidents that have happened to horses known to you.

1.

2.

With the benefit of hindsight, what steps could have been taken to prevent these accidents from occurring?

ESTABLISHING EMERGENCIES AND EQUINE FIRST AID

When, despite our best intentions, accidents do occur, it is important to react in a prompt and appropriate manner. Initially, the most crucial thing is to determine whether what has happened constitutes an emergency. Dictionary definitions of an emergency include: 'A sudden happening which makes it necessary to act without delay' and 'A sudden state or condition needing immediate treatment'. In equestrian terms, a true emergency, needing immediate attention, would include any condition:

- Where there is an immediate threat to the horse's life, e.g. colic, difficult foaling, dehydration.

- Where, although the injury itself does not threaten the horse's life, the implications of the injury may permanently incapacitate the horse, e.g. a puncture wound in the foot or on a joint; a fracture within a joint.

- Where delaying treatment may seriously compromise the successful outcome (the **golden period** of wound healing is explained in Chapter 2.)

- Where delay of treatment will prolong the horse's suffering, e.g. laminitis.

The term 'first aid' is commonly thought of as meaning 'dealing promptly with relatively minor injuries' and hopefully, in many cases, that will be all that is necessary. Good first aid may be so successful that further treatment is not necessary. (The shorter the time between the injury occurring and the administration of appropriate first aid, the more likely it is that complications, infection, etc. will be avoided.) However, in essence, first aid means 'the first assistance that can be given' and, in some situations, this may mean acting to limit or prevent the deterioration of a very serious condition, until such time as top-rate professional help becomes available. Whether 'minor' or 'major' first aid is necessary, one of its chief aims is always to relieve the horse's suffering and discomfort.

ITQ 2 Give three examples of an equine emergency.

1.

2.

3.

ITQ 3 What are the main aims of first aid?

1.
2.
3.
4.

THE EQUINE FIRST AID KIT

Every horse owner must have at least a basic first aid kit. Larger yards, dealing with larger numbers of horses, will need more than one first aid kit. Keep the kits separately so that they are easily accessible from different points of the yard. Also, keep the vet's phone number displayed near all telephones on the yard so that the vet can be contacted quickly without having to search for the number. The vet's phone number should also be entered on yard staff's mobile phones.

The equine first aid kit should be:
- Stored in a suitable container – a plastic box with a lid is ideal.
- Clearly labelled.
- Kept clean and regularly updated. All medications in the first aid box must be discarded once they have exceeded their use-by date.
- Easily accessible at all times (other than to unauthorized people, e.g. children).

Important constituents of a first aid kit are explained in the following sub-sections. A smaller kit containing items likely to be needed when travelling or at an event should be kept in the lorry.

Dressings

Melolin dressings – a perforated film, non-adherent, absorbent dressing which absorbs excessive exudate (defined in Chapter 2) from the wound without drying it out. It also allows the wound to 'breathe'.

Conformable polymeric foam dressings – the outer membrane provides a low-adherent wound contact layer and is perforated to allow exudate to pass into the interior of the dressing. Foam dressings also cushion the wound.

Carbon/silver impregnated dressings – help promote wound closure and cleansing by absorbing bacteria. Mainly used in chronic/infected wounds.

Soffban – a non-woven padding material which provides cushioning and protection. Used as an additional layer between the wound dressing and other padding.

Animalintex poultices – these ready-to-use poultices contain a mild antiseptic, boric acid, to promote healing and a natural poultice agent, tragacinth. They are ideal for puncture wounds of the foot or to draw exudate out from an infected wound and they can be used hot, cold or dry.

Cotton wool – this should not be used as a dressing as it sticks to the wound. However, busy yards should keep a large supply of rolls of cotton wool in case a horse sustains a limb fracture. Several rolls of cotton wool are needed to provide padding when splinting a fracture or applying pressure bandages.

Tube-grip – an elasticated tube-bandage which is very useful for holding dressings in place on the limbs, in particular on joints where some mobility is needed.

Gamgee – this provides extra padding and support when used underneath bandages. As it is not sterile, it should not be used directly on a wound. Instead, Melolin should be placed against the wound. However, Gamgee can be cut into different size swabs and used to clean wounds in conjunction with an anti-bacterial solution. This is preferable to using cotton wool, which can leave fibres in the wound.

Assorted conforming crepe bandages – including support bandages, e.g. Bonner bandages. Bandages are needed for support purposes and to hold dressings in place. At least ten rolls of elastic gauze bandages are needed for initial fracture treatment.

Vetrap (cohesive) bandages – cohesive bandages are invaluable for holding dressings in place. They are particularly useful for protecting poultices on the foot and on the limbs.

Cold bandages – these include gel packs which can be kept in the freezer, ready to use.

Cleansing, Antiseptic and Topical Agents

Topical agents are those applied to the surface of the body, as opposed to being injected, ingested or applied through invasive surgery.

Saline solution – physiological saline (a sterile solution of sodium chloride that has an equal concentration of solutes to body fluids) is the best solution for flushing fresh wounds. Saline solution can be made up using 1 teaspoon of salt to 0.57 litres (1 pint) of warm, previously boiled, water – or it can be purchased in small packs.

Hibiscrub – chlorhexidene gluconate in an alcoholic solution – is an antiseptic effective against bacteria and should be well diluted in water (0.05% solution). Hibiscrub is effective as it binds to cells.

Pevidine – this is an iodine-based antiseptic cleansing agent which must be well diluted (0.1–1% solution). Strong solutions can cause tissue damage and nerve damage, and thus interfere with healing. Iodine solutions tend to be used for wounds of the foot and are not the agent of choice for broken skin.

Antibiotic cream, gel or spray – in the early stages of healing a wound should be kept moist, so a cream or gel is ideal. Dermisol is a healing cream which can be used beneath a dry dressing. Fucidin or Protocon ointments are valuable when treating cracked heels or mud fever.

Wound hydrogel – water-soluble gels such as Intrasite Gel, Nugel, Derma-gel and Vetalintex – rehydrate the wound and provide the optimum environment for healing.

Petroleum jelly – can be used to pack the heels prior to cold hosing treatment to prevent cracking, applied to abrasions to help prevent contamination from flies and debris and used as a thermometer lubricant.

Hardware

Clean bucket – for scrubbing out the feet, etc.

Clean plastic bowl – to prepare cleansing solutions, poultices, etc.

Plastic spray gun (the sort used to spray house plants). Ideal for spraying cleansing solution onto awkward wounds.

Plastic syringes – if sealed, these provide a sterile method of cleansing and flushing a wound. Saline solution can be squirted into the wound (*without* the needle!).

Veterinary thermometer – digital thermometers are easy to use and safe.

Surgical scissors – rounded and blunt-ended for clipping away hair from the site of a wound. Straight, sharp scissors are needed for cutting dressings and Gamgee.

Bandage/electrical tape – used to help an adhesive bandage keep a dressing in place.

Duct/gaffer tape – useful as the outer protective layer of a foot poultice.

Twitch – used to restrain a horse if necessary during treatment.

Tweezers – for removing thorns.

Stethoscope – to listen to the heart.

Hoof testers – used to squeeze the hoof to test for pain within the foot.

Poultice/hoof boot – a tough protective boot that fits over the foot. Can be used temporarily when a shoe is lost, or to hold a poultice in place.

ITQ 4 What are the following used for?

a. Melolin

b. Pevidine

CHAPTER SUMMARY

You must always bear in mind that the horse is very much a 'fright, flight, fight' animal. Inherently, the flight response is very strong – the horse has survived to date using flight as his main defence. As the horse takes flight he tends to move at speed with little regard for the safety of his hastily chosen path. Unfortunately, this renders horses susceptible to injury.

This chapter has dealt mainly with accident prevention. As with every undesirable incident in life 'prevention is better than cure' but, whilst precautions can and must be taken to improve safety, it's not possible to prevent every accident from occurring. Therefore, having looked at accident prevention, we've also looked at what may constitute an emergency and the contents of the first aid kit. Next, we move onto discuss what to do when the horse sustains an injury.

CHAPTER 2

WOUND MANAGEMENT

The aims and objectives of this chapter are to explain:

- The different types of wound.
- The stages of wound healing and the factors that affect healing.
- The differences between arterial, venous and capillary haemorrhage.
- The factors leading to the natural arrest of bleeding.
- The first aid measures that can be used to stop bleeding.
- The causes and treatment of haematoma, oedema, abscess and inflammation.
- The main principles of wound management.
- The wounds that are potentially life-threatening to the horse.
- The range of dressings and bandaging techniques used in the treatment of serious wounds.
- The types, causes and signs of fractures (as these are some of the most serious types of wound).
- The first aid treatment of a horse with a suspected fracture.

Because of the soft tissue trauma associated with them, fractures and their management are viewed and discussed as wounds. (Some types of fracture involve some of the most serious types of wound.)

TYPES OF WOUND

We will start by looking at the different types of wounds, their likely causes, methods of healing and treatments. Wounds are either **open** or **closed**.

OPEN WOUNDS

Wounds to the skin can be caused by cutting, puncturing or tearing. The injury may involve damage to or the loss of epidermal tissue, epidermis and upper dermis. The whole of the epidermis and dermis may be involved and, in the case of deep wounds, the underlying tissues may also be damaged or lost.

Superficial wounds (grazes/abrasions) involve loss of the epidermis or the epidermis and superficial layer of the dermis. Provided a superficial wound does not become infected, it should heal in approximately ten days. Full-thickness skin wounds are slow to heal unless the edges of the wound can be bought together. If the wound cannot be closed for some reason, healing occurs through wound contraction, repair and regeneration. These processes are discussed later in this chapter.

The healing of **deep wounds** can be complicated by the formation of scar tissue. This is also discussed further on.

Open wounds can also be categorized as follows:

- **Incised or clean-cut wounds** – caused by a sharp object such as a knife or piece of glass, these have clean edges and, depending on location, should heal quickly and simply. The amount of bleeding will depend upon the depth of the wound and whether blood vessels are involved. There may be damage to underlying muscle.

- **Lacerated or tear wounds** – these can occur as a result of entanglement with barbed wire or snagging on a nail or other protrusion. Tear wounds have uneven, torn edges, often resulting in flaps of skin. There is often bruising associated with a tear wound. The level of bleeding will depend upon the damage caused to underlying blood vessels.

- **Puncture wounds** – these have a small point of entry which is difficult to see, often caused by a nail, wood splinter, piece of wire, etc. The wound can become infected as the object causing the puncture may introduce bacteria, dirt, etc. into the deeper tissues. Puncture wounds must heal from the inside out to prevent infection from developing and becoming trapped within the wound. This usually involves poulticing, e.g. with Animalintex, to draw out the infection.

It is important that a horse who has sustained a puncture wound is protected against **tetanus** as the tetanus bacteria, *Clostridium tetani* are present in the soil and may find their way into the wound. Within the wound these anaerobic bacteria multiply and release the tetanus toxin which paralyses the central nervous system. If the horse's vaccination status is unknown, the vet will give a tetanus anti-toxin immediately.

A puncture wound on a joint is potentially very serious, as infection within a joint can lead to permanent unsoundness. If there is a suspicion of infection the vet may prescribe antibiotics, to be added to the feed and/or by intravenous injection.

ITQ 5 State two of the main complications that may occur with a puncture wound.

1.

2.

ITQ 6 What steps must be taken to avoid these complications?

CLOSED WOUNDS

- **Bruises or contused wounds** – these result from a blow such as a kick or a fall. Haemorrhage (bleeding) and **oedema** (fluid-filled swelling) occurs beneath the skin. Certain contusions will result in formation of a **haematoma** (blood-filled swelling). Underlying bone may be also damaged, e.g. after a kick. Stepping on a sharp stone can cause a bruised sole. A severe bruise accompanied by skin damage is normally referred to as a contusion.

- **Abscesses**. An abscess is defined as a cavity containing dead cells, bacteria and exudate and can be caused by the presence of foreign bodies, bacterial or fungal infection or migrating parasitic larvae. An abscess may form and burst quickly, i.e. it is acute, or it may develop slowly and not burst until it reaches the surface of the body. Abscesses can occur in all tissues of the body; a relatively common example is pus in the foot.

- **Tendon injury** – depending upon the nature and extent of the injury, the tendon fibres are torn or stretched, which may lead to haemorrhage within the tendon. Fluids seep through from adjacent tissues resulting in a hot, painful swelling.

- **Limb fracture** – a bone may fracture when subjected to a particular force or stress. In the horse, this may occur as a result of a kick, fall, blow, putting a foot down a hole whilst cantering or some similar accident. (While fractures are commonly closed wounds, some types, i.e. compound fractures, have an open element. Fractures are explained in more detail later in this chapter.)

FACTORS AFFECTING WOUND HEALING

Wound healing is affected by:

- **The site of the wound**. Wounds, even large/spectacular ones, on the large muscle masses where the skin is relatively loose, can heal very quickly and effectively, leaving minimal scarring. However, a small, innocuous-looking wound on a lower limb (especially if a joint is involved) can be troublesome and difficult to heal. Permanent damage can be caused by a puncture wound in the heel region of the foot as the navicular bursa may be infected – in fact, with potentially fatal consequences. Joints are also susceptible to infection which, again, can cause permanent damage. Any wound on a joint must be considered serious and in need of urgent veterinary attention.

- **The initial treatment**. If a wound needs stitching this should be carried out as soon as possible after injury, before the area becomes swollen or infected. Wounds are always contaminated but have what is called the '**golden period**' in which suturing or stapling can be carried out success-fully before infection sets in. The golden period never exceeds 4 hours – in the horse it is much shorter. During this time the wound is only contaminated, not infected.

- **Infection**. Infection occurs as a result of increasing numbers of contaminating organisms (bacteria), the presence of organic matter (debris) and loss of blood supply within the wound. Infection causes further tissue damage, discharge and inflammation, thus impairing the healing process.

- **Blood supply to the wound**. A healthy blood supply is needed for effective healing. Tissue damage can result in impaired blood supply, which will affect the amount of oxygen arriving at the site. Lack of oxygen will lead to tissue death – this is termed **necrosis**. Necrotic tissue will impair healing as well as preventing topically applied antibiotics from reaching the bacteria within the wound.

- **Hydration and warmth**. The horse's body consists of approximately 70 per cent water. In the early stages of healing the wound should be kept moist and warm through being covered with a dressing and bandage. If a wound is left open to the air in the early stages it becomes dehydrated, which causes the tissues to become devitalized. This compromises healing.

- **Soft tissue damage**. Bruising and haematomas (blood sacs) will interfere with the healing process.

- **Vitamin deficiency**. Vitamin K is involved in the formation of the blood-clotting protein, fibrinogen. Collagen production is influenced by the presence of Vitamin C. This affects healing as skin is comprised mainly of collagen, a fibrous protein.

ITQ 7 What are the following?

a. Oedema.

b. Haematoma.

c. Necrosis.

ITQ 8 Give a definition of an abscess.

ITQ 9 What is meant by the 'golden period' of a wound?

ITQ 10 Why should wounds on a joint be considered potentially very serious?

ITQ 11 Why should a wound be kept warm and moist in the early stages of healing?

THE HEALING PROCESS

There are two defined methods by which wound healing takes place:

1. **First (or primary) intention healing**. This involves the edges of the wound being held together, knitting and subsequently healing quickly and effectively. This is the case in surgical wounds or clean, incised wounds where no infection or tissue loss occurs and the wound can be held together by sutures or staples. This type of healing generally results in minimal scarring.

2. **Second intention healing**. This occurs when there has been loss of tissue, excessive movement of the wound, or infection. One or a combination of these factors prevents the wound edges from being held together and/or knitting together, which delays healing.

    The wound has to fill with new tissue, **granulation tissue**, before new skin grows over the wound. This often results in the formation of **proud flesh** and often an unsightly scar.

ITQ 12 What is meant by primary intention wound healing?

ITQ 13

a. What is meant by second intention wound healing?

b. Give another name for scar tissue.

THE STAGES OF WOUND HEALING
First Stage: the Traumatic Inflammatory (Defensive) Phase

Damage to the tissues initiates an **inflammatory response**. The inflammatory process occurs in two phases.

1. **The immediate response** (within 20 minutes) whereby blood flow to the area is increased and plasma leaks into the surrounding tissue. Externally, this can be seen as redness (depending upon site and coat colour) and felt as heat (inflammation).

2. **The delayed response**. Externally, this shows as swelling and pain. The leakage of plasma continues; blood flow through the affected area is impeded – although bleeding into surrounding tissue may occur. Specialized white blood cells invade the area.

The inflammatory response can be seen:
1. When disease is caused by infection (e.g. strangles).
2. When injury has occurred in tissue such as tendon or bone.
3. Where a wound has been sustained.

Chemical messengers from the damaged cells stimulate undamaged cells which release the chemical substances **bradykinin** and **histamine**. These increase the permeability of the capillary walls, allowing plasma, white blood cells and platelets to leak onto the surface of the wound. This is termed **exudate**.

The amount of exudate will depend upon the nature of the injury. If extensive damage has occurred the capillaries will be over-stimulated, resulting in excessive exudate, swelling and pain. Within the exudate will be agents concerned with blood clotting, debris removal and fighting infection (the last two of which take place mainly in the following stages of healing).

Blood clotting takes place through the following process. The blood platelets release the enzyme **thrombokinase**, which reacts with a substance called **prothrombin**, resulting in the formation of **thrombin**. Thrombin acts on **fibrinogen** (a blood protein formed in the liver, which circulates in the plasma). The combination of fibrinogen and thrombin results in the formation of **fibrin** strands. These strands form a mesh, in which red blood cells get trapped; the mesh then contracts to form a **clot**. Serum escapes from the clot – this is seen as a clear yellow fluid. Initially, the clot is thick and gelatinous, but its outer surface then hardens to form a **scab**.

Second Stage: the Destructive Phase (Debris Removal)

In response to messages sent by the damaged cells, specialized white blood cells (**leucocytes**) move to the injured area.

The leucocytes concerned with defence against infection are known as **neutrophils**. They are also called **polymorphonuclear leucocytes (PMNs)**, because they can change shape as they move through tissue. They originate

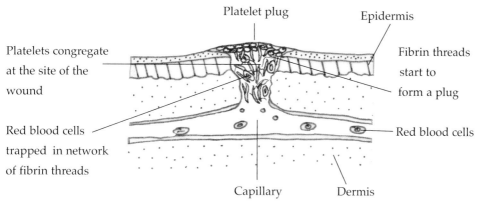

Platelet plug

Epidermis

Platelets congregate at the site of the wound

Fibrin threads start to form a plug

Red blood cells trapped in network of fibrin threads

Red blood cells

Capillary

Dermis

Figure 2 Blood clotting

in the bone marrow and engulf and destroy invading bacteria in a process known as **phagocytosis**. The PMN 'recognizes' the invading bacterium as foreign and adheres to its surface. It then engulfs the bacterium and kills it.

After approximately eight hours white blood cells originating in the lymphatic system (**monocytes**) move into the area where they become **macrophages** – specialized cells with the specific task of clearing away dead tissue or debris. The macrophages ingest and destroy the debris – this is referred to as the **destructive phase** of wound healing. Basically, the macrophages are clearing the way, prior to the formation of new healthy tissue.

Third Stage: the Reconstructive Phase

Macrophages also stimulate the production of fibre-forming cells or **fibroblasts**. Fibroblasts are responsible for the formation of **collagen**, the body's main supportive structural protein. At this stage fibroblasts make a network of disorganized collagen fibrils.

Granulation tissue (or **proud flesh**) is formed. This consists of loops of newly formed capillaries supported by collagen fibres, filling the wound and covering its surface. Generally, the greater the inflammation, the more proud flesh will form. Excessive proud flesh is undesirable as it produces an unsightly scar, can affect limb function (especially if near a joint) and prevents new skin growth from covering the wound. Therefore, inflammation needs to be reduced and controlled. The method for doing this is dealt with in Chapter 3.

Movement of the edges of the wound at this stage can compromise the healing process. Therefore the wound must be immobilized to give it the best chances of healing. Box rest and bandaging can be useful in this respect.

Fourth stage: the Maturation Phase (Epithelialization and Contraction)

As the granulation tissue matures it is referred to as a **scar**. The new scar tissue is highly vascular (contains many capillaries), resulting in a red colouration. As the granulation tissue develops it contracts, pulling the edges of the wound closer together. Contraction reduces the size of the wound.

Scar tissue becomes stronger as the collagen fibres enlarge and become reorganized. As the tissue matures its vascularity decreases. It changes to avascular tissue (i.e. with no blood supply), which is a pale whiteish colour. Whilst the scar tissue becomes stronger, it never regains the full strength of undamaged tissue. Eventually the scar reduces.

MULTIPLE CHOICE QUESTIONS
(THERE MAY BE MORE THAN ONE CORRECT ANSWER)

ITQ 14 The combination of thrombin and fibrinogen results in the formation of:

1. Prothrombin?
2. Fibrin?
3. Thrombokinase?
4. Exudate?

ITQ 15 The blood cells concerned with defence against infection are:

1. Monocytes?
2. Platelets?
3. Neutrophils?
4. PMNs?

ITQ 16 The specialized cells which clear debris away from the site of a wound:

1. Originate in the bone marrow?
2. Are called neutrophils?
3. Originate in the lymphatic system?

ITQ 17 What is phagocytosis?

ITQ 18

a. What are the cells called that produce collagen?

b. Which vitamin influences the formation of collagen?

WOUND MANAGEMENT

A serious wound will need veterinary attention. If a joint is affected, the wound is bleeding seriously and/or looks as though it will need stitching, call the vet. This should be done as soon as is practical, but it will help the vet if a reasonably concise and accurate description of the injury can be given.

The following are the sequential steps in wound management.

1. Controlling Bleeding

Bleeding must be controlled to prevent excessive blood loss. The type of bleeding can be identified as follows:

- **Venous bleeding**. If bleeding is from a vein, the blood flow will be slow and continual. The blood is deoxygenated and therefore dark in colour.

- **Arterial bleeding**. If an artery is damaged the blood will escape in spurts as it is pumped out under pressure by the heart. Arterial blood is oxygenated so is bright red in colour.

The following methods are used to control bleeding:

Pressure – can be applied directly by holding the edges of the wound together and pressing firmly. Initially, you may not have first aid equipment with you so you will need to improvise by using your sweatshirt or sock as a pressure pad in the first instance. When you are able to do so, apply a clean dressing to the wound and hold it firmly in place until the bleeding stops.

If the injury is on a limb, a wad of clean material can be bandaged firmly over the wound using a cotton bandage. If the bleeding is profuse or blood seeps through, do not remove the bandage – apply another bandage over the top and leave it in place until the vet arrives.

Once the bleeding has stopped the bandage must be removed. If left in place too long, it may interfere with the normal circulation of blood, resulting in skin or tendon necrosis.

Tourniquets should not be used as they can cause complications and make bleeding worse by interfering with the venous return of blood.

Cold hosing. If the wound is not bleeding very much, gentle hosing with cold water will cause the capillaries to constrict, thereby stemming the bleeding.

> ITQ 19
>
> a. How can you tell whether bleeding is venous or arterial?
>
> b. What can be done to stem severe bleeding?

2. Cleansing

The following help with the cleansing process.

Hosing. In addition to encouraging capillary restriction, gentle hosing is an effective way of washing the wound and surrounding coat, especially if it is dirty. Do not use high pressure, as particles of debris may be pushed deeper into the wound and blood vessels and cells may be damaged or blood clots disturbed, causing bleeding.

Clip the hair surrounding the wound if it will make it easier to see and clean. Curved scissors or clippers can be used. Pack the wound with KY jelly or Intrasite Gel before clipping to prevent hair clippings from contaminating it. (This must be done after any hosing, otherwise the gel would interfere with the washing process.)

Wash your hands. Before you start to clean the wound more carefully, you must wash your hands to reduce the risk of introducing infection. For large wounds you should wear disposable gloves.

Antiseptic washes. Once the wound has been hosed and the surrounding hair clipped, the gauze packing can be removed and the wound should be flushed through. Fresh wounds do not need to be washed with antiseptic solutions. Flush through with sterile saline solution made from 1 teaspoon salt to 0.57 litres (1 pint) of warm, previously boiled water, using a plastic syringe or hand pump.

Older or contaminated wounds should be flushed with 0.5% solution of Hibiscrub.

Swabs to apply the washes can be made from Gamgee; cotton wool tends to stick to large wounds, although it is satisfactory for use on small wounds. Gamgee swabs are thus more effective for larger wounds. Soak the swabs in the solution and, starting in the middle of the wound, wipe out towards the edges to prevent any dirt from the coat being introduced into the wound. Use each swab once only to reduce contamination.

Once the wound is clean, do not pack it with wound powder or cream before the vet arrives. He needs to see the wound clearly. The wound can be covered with a clean dressing while waiting for the vet.

3. Debridement

Once the wound has been thoroughly cleaned it may be necessary to debride it. This involves the removal of embedded debris, dead or damaged tissue and tags of skin. If left, these would interfere with healing and lead to infection. Depending upon the size and site of the wound it may be necessary to sedate the horse and use a local anaesthetic while the vet uses tissue forceps, scissors and a scalpel to debride the wound.

4. Suturing (stitching)

The wound should be sutured as early as possible to avoid the risk of infection. Suturing will only be possible if there is sufficient loose skin to draw the edges of the wound together. Subcutaneous and deeper tissues can be stitched together using absorbable sutures, before the skin is then stitched. Sutures are normally left in place for around ten days. Staples can be used as a quick alternative to sutures.

5. Drainage

Certain types of wounds will need drainage to prevent a build-up of fluid and debris, e.g. puncture wounds and wounds where tissue loss has left a hole. Plastic or latex drains may be sutured into the wound, allowing exudate and debris to drain away from the wound to the outside. Alternatively, a small opening may be made in the skin at the lowest point of the wound. Care must be taken that the opening or drains do not become contaminated, since this could lead to infection.

> **ITQ 20 What strength should the solutions be for:**
>
> a. Hibiscrub?
>
> b. Saline solution?

> **ITQ 21 Why is debridement of the wound sometimes necessary?**

> **ITQ 22**
>
> a. What is proud flesh?
>
> b. Why is excessive proud flesh undesirable?

6. Dressing

The actual dressings have various functions:
- Preventing contamination of the site of the wound.
- Protecting the site from further damage.
- Absorbing exudates.
- Maintaining a moist environment.
- Maintaining the temperature at the site of the wound/preventing excessive variation.
- Promote gaseous exchange.
- Promoting healing.

Subject to the vet's advice, the wound should be kept moist to promote healing. Hydrogels ensure a moist environment and can be applied prior to the application of a dressing, unless the dressing used is designed to meet this requirement.

The dressings used should be sterile (or at least very clean) and non-adhesive, e.g. Melolin. The dressing will allow air to circulate, thus improving the supply of oxygen to the wound, and absorb excessive exudate (which impairs the supply of oxygen within the wound). At the same time it prevents the wound from drying out, ensuring that the white blood cells within the exudate can perform their task of fighting infection effectively. Conformable foam dressings are ideal and different shaped dressings can be purchased, ensuring adequate coverage and protection.

Some dressings have a moist surface and are impregnated with antibiotic. These should be used with care, subject to veterinary advice, to ensure that the horse is not allergic to the impregnated antibiotic, and that it does not compromise the action of any other drugs administered in other ways. If these safeguards are adhered to, these dressings are suitable for use in the early stages of healing as a moist wound surface encourages epithelial migration (granulation tissue migrating across the wound surface). They should not however, be used over a prolonged period as keeping the wound moist for *too long* will encourage the formation of excessive granulation tissue (proud flesh).

Animalintex poultices are made from gauze and wool, impregnated with boracic powder and they can be used as a dry dressing to aid wound healing, or cold and wet to reduce inflammation, or warm and wet to draw out infection.

BANDAGING
Benefits of bandaging

Wounds may need to be bandaged for the following reasons:

- **To secure the dressing**. Bandaging holds a dressing in place to keep the wound clean and prevent it from drying out at first.

- **To apply pressure**. This will control and reduce swelling.

- **Moisture retention**. Bandaging helps to keep the wound moist initially, which promotes circulation. This ensures a good oxygen supply to the wound. Although bandaging reduces the wound's uptake of atmospheric oxygen, wound dehydration leads to decreased circulation, which deprives the wound of the internal oxygen source.

- **Immobilization**. Bandaging helps to immobilize the wound site and control swelling, which protects it from distortion. Good bandaging provides a stable support for the migration of new skin cells across the wound. The wound surface is distorted by movement, swelling or trauma, in which case healing is delayed.

- **Limitation of proud flesh**. While the bandage must not be applied too tightly, slight pressure reduces the development of proud flesh, so reduces scarring.

- **Retention of body temperature**. The optimum temperature for wound healing is approximately 86 °F. Should the temperature fall below 68 °F circulation is impaired resulting in reduced blood flow to the area.

Bandaging Technique
LAYERS

A properly constructed bandage consists of three layers:

1. **Primary layer**. This is the dressing which is in direct contact with the wound.

2. **Secondary layer**. This can be a layer of cotton wool or Gamgee. Cotton wool is useful because it is soft, easily moulded, absorbent and conforms to the shape of the affected area. It is also less expensive than Gamgee. An alternative to cotton wool is a product called 'Soffban'; an absorbent orthopaedic padding in the form of a roll which is applied like a bandage. It is useful for holding dressings in place prior to the Gamgee being applied.
   The functions of the secondary layer are:
   - To absorb exudate and keep it away from the wound surface.
   - To distribute the pressure of the bandage over the whole area.
   - To provide a degree of splintage to the area, helping to immobilize the wound.

Sufficient padding should be used to absorb all of the exudate and should be changed when saturated.

3. **Tertiary layer**. This outer layer secures the primary and secondary layer to the wound and protects them from the external environment. Tension is applied to each wrap in order to compress the secondary layer, which helps to increase rigidity and distributes the pressure evenly over the area. The tertiary layer normally consists of an elastic gauze bandage and/or an elasticated self-adherent cohesive (Vetrap) bandage. Electrical tape may be used to secure the end of the cohesive bandage.

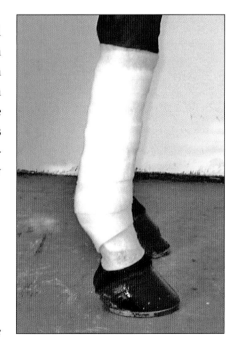

Figure 3 Bandaging – Soffban holding a dressing in place

CONSIDERATIONS WHEN BANDAGING

Important considerations when bandaging are:

- The bandage and padding must be flat, not lumpy or wrinkled, as this will cause pressure points.

- Bandage in the same direction that the padding overlaps, e.g. if the padding overlaps left over right, wrap the bandage around the limb from left to right (anticlockwise). This prevents the padding from becoming ridged and uneven.

- Start bandaging in the middle, working first down and then up. This provides security and helps prevent the bandage from slipping. It is also thought that bandaging upwards helps prevent fluid filling in the limb.

- The whole of the lower limb should be bandaged – any unbandaged area would be prone to filling.

- Ensure that about 2.5 cm (1 inch) of padding is left exposed at the top and bottom to prevent pressure sores and restriction of circulation.

- Each wrap should overlap the previous turn by about half the width of the bandage for even distribution of pressure.

- Never bandage too tightly, as the circulation may be impaired.

- The tertiary layer may be wrapped in a circular, spiral or figure of eight pattern.

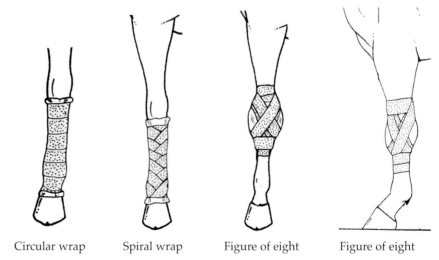

| Circular wrap | Spiral wrap | Figure of eight | Figure of eight |

Figure 4 Methods of bandaging – the tertiary layer

METHODS

Methods of bandaging are:

Circular wrap. This provides maximal 'hold' – it prevents slippage provided it is applied at the correct tension.

Spiral wrap. This method is useful where a high level of support is needed, e.g. to prevent over-extension of the fetlock joint after tendon or ligament injury.

Figure of eight. This method is used on the knee and hock to avoid the concentration of pressure on the accessory carpal bone and os calcis. It also helps to immobilize the joint, which promotes healing. The padding should be loose in the region of these bones. Adhesive bandages are ideal for figure of eight wraps as they do not slip. The bandage can overlap the padding, contacting the coat to seal the area. The bandage must not be pulled tight on the coat as this will cause irritation and constriction.

The figure of eight can be positioned according to the site of the injury. If it is necessary to limit movement of the knee or hock, the figure of eight can be across the front of the joint. If the dressing is on the knee, the figure of eight should be on the lateral aspect. It should not pass across the back of the knee or hock, as pressure will be exerted on the accessory carpal bone and os calcis.

SUPPORTING AND AUXILIARY BANDAGES

A **support bandage** should be applied to the whole lower limb to prevent filling and provide support. A support bandage must also be applied to the *sound* limb as this will be bearing additional weight while the horse favours the injured limb.

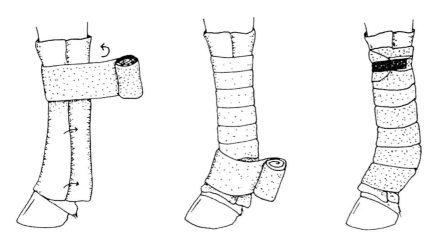

Figure 5 Applying a support bandage

Tubular bandages (commonly known by names such as tube-grip) can be purchased from the chemist. These will fit over the knee or hock to hold a dressing in place. One advantage of tubular bandages is that an opening can be cut in the bandage in the area over the back of the knee or hock, preventing excessive pressure at these points. You do not need to remove the bandage every time you change the dressing – simply roll the lower edge of the bandage up while you clean the wound.

The tubular bandage in Figure 6 is held in place at the top by Flexoplast, a highly adhesive bandage. The bottom of the tubular bandage is sealed with Flexoplast to prevent bedding from working up the bandage and to prevent slippage.

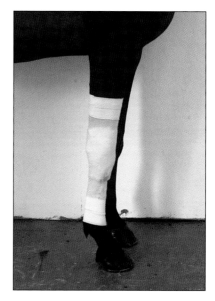

Figure 6 A tubular bandage

Zip-up (Pressage) bandages for the knee and hock are designed to exert an even pressure and are useful for holding dressings in place.

ITQ 23 In terms of wound healing, list the four benefits of bandaging.

1.

2.

3.

4.

ITQ 24 Name the three layers of a well-constructed bandage and give the functions of each.

1.

2.

3.

Care of Bandages

The frequency with which a bandage should be changed will depend upon the advice given by the vet and the nature of the wound or injury; it need not be daily. It will need to be changed when:

- The padding is soiled with exudate.
- The bandage and padding have become badly soiled externally, e.g. with faeces.
- There has been slippage of bandage and/or padding, or disruption by the horse.
- A poultice needs to be replaced (normally done twice daily in the early stages, then once daily).

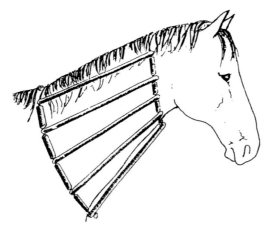

If the horse is interfering with the bandage he may need to wear a neck cradle or bib which will prevent him from taking hold of the bandages. Alternatively, dab bitter aloes (or a similar product) on the bandage.

Figure 7 A cradle

Provided the bandages are being monitored frequently, they can stay in place as long as they are functional.

ITQ 25 When bandaging, what can be done to ensure that the tension and distribution of pressure are even?

TREATMENT OF PUNCTURE WOUNDS

Puncture wounds of the foot or on a joint must be treated as potentially very serious.

Punctured Sole

This is often caused as a result of the horse standing on a sharp object, such as a nail. Any penetration in or around the frog requires immediate veterinary attention. Punctures of the middle third of the frog are the most serious and often require surgery as the navicular bursa may be punctured and infected.

SIGNS

Varying degrees of lameness will be seen. In some cases the horse will be fracture-lame, i.e. non-weightbearing. (This is very serious and warrants immediate veterinary attention). If the puncture goes undetected for any length of time there will almost invariably be infection within the foot. An abscess will form and, if the important structures of the foot – the pedal bone and navicular bursa – are involved, it may result in permanent unsoundness.

(Abnormal heat in the foot is an indication of infection, especially if accompanied by lameness.)

TREATMENT

If the penetrating object (normally a nail) is still in the foot, try to prevent the horse from moving around and pushing it in further. If the vet is known to have a portable X-ray machine it may be useful to leave the object *in situ* pending the vet's arrival, so that the degree of penetration and damage can be assessed. Discuss this during the initial phone call to the vet. Also, if the penetration looks severe, the horse may need to be admitted to an equine hospital for the removal of the object and antibiotic therapy to prevent infection.

If the object is no longer in the foot, it will be necessary to find the point of penetration by scrubbing the foot. Details such as point of entry, length of object, depth and direction of penetration should be recorded as fully as possible, to assist the vet and, if the penetrating object can be found, this should also be retained.

If the penetration seems at all serious, veterinary assistance should certainly be sought. Even if the injury appears minor, should there be any doubt about the status of the horse's tetanus vaccinations, the vet should still be called, to give a tetanus antitoxin injection. Veterinary administration of antibiotics may also be necessary to counter any infection. The vet may also open the hole and pare away a little of the sole to allow the escape of pus.

Poulticing is an established method of cleaning wounds and drawing out infection. Whilst an attending vet may apply an initial poultice, it is useful to know how to do this in order to repeat the treatment. To apply a poultice you will need:

— Antiseptic wash (Pevidine or similar).
— Very hot water.
— Animalintex poultice (ready-cut into a square, although hoof-shaped Animalintex can be purchased.)
— A piece of polythene sheeting.
— Gamgee or Soffban.
— Self-adhesive bandage.
— Hoof or poultice boot or duct tape.

1. Pick out and thoroughly scrub the foot with Pevidine solution (it is at this point that an object still in the foot would be removed, if it was considered safe to do so).

2. Soak the ready-cut square of Animalintex in nearly boiling water. Wring out the excess water and place the impregnated side of the poultice to the sole of the foot.

3. Press in place firmly and cover with a piece of polythene, then a large square of Gamgee, or encase in Soffban. Completely bandage the whole foot using an adhesive bandage.

4. Either cover the sole with duct tape to protect the adhesive bandage or put on the hoof/poultice boot. This layer prevents the bandage from becoming worn and moisture from the stable floor, e.g. urine and faeces, being absorbed into the dressing.

5. Bandage the lower limb with a stable bandage and padding such as Gamgee. This supports the limb and prevents filling. Bandage the sound leg to give extra support and prevent filling.

Poultices should be changed once daily or as instructed by the vet. Once the infection has been completely drawn out, the hole can be plugged with a small piece of cotton wool soaked in Pevidine to prevent contamination. The farrier may shoe using a pad to protect the damaged are, but only once all risk of infection has gone.

1. Animalintex

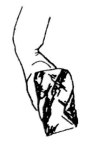

2. Polythene

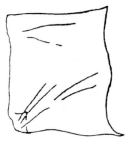

3. Gamgee

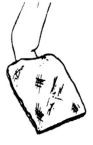

4. Adhesive bandage

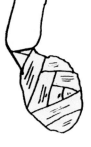

5. Hoof boot or duct tape

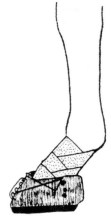

Figure 8 Poulticing the foot

Puncture Wounds of the Skin

Puncture wounds of the skin are often caused by thorns and can lead to infection. Poulticing can be an effective method of removing the object and any subsequent infection. If the object is embedded in the flesh, call the vet to remove it – do not dig around yourself as you will be likely to force it in further and cause contamination of the wound.

Puncture wounds on joints are very serious. Apart from the risk of joint fluid leaking, the greatest risk is that of infection. This can be disastrous, leading to permanent loss of use of the horse, so the vet should be consulted immediately.

A wound on a joint must be thoroughly cleaned and then covered to prevent contamination. It must be kept scrupulously clean. The vet will administer antibiotics to reduce the risk of infection.

If there is a suspicion that the joint is infected the horse will need to be admitted to a veterinary hospital. A sample of joint fluid will be taken to ascertain the presence of infection. If infected, the joint will need to be flushed and treated aggressively to save the horse. There is still a risk that some horses may not regain soundness.

Key Points to Remember with Puncture Wounds

- Because of the risk of damage to internal structures, puncture wounds can be very serious, with the possibility of permanent damage. Consult the vet immmediately. Early aggressive treatment may make the difference between success and failure.

- Even the smallest puncture wound may prove fatal in certain circumstances. In particular, the horse must be up to date with his tetanus vaccinations. The anaerobic bacteria *Clostridium tetani* are present in the soil. If the bacteria enter a puncture wound they are then in the ideal environment for reproduction and multiplication. The toxin released by the bacteria is usually fatal.

- If any horse is severely and rapidly lame (i.e. in less than 24 hours) following a puncture wound to a limb, call the vet.

- The wound must heal from the inside out to prevent infection developing within.

ITQ 26

a. Why are puncture wounds potentially very serious?

b. What are the main aims when treating such a wound?

ITQ 27 How should a puncture wound on a joint be treated?

Penetration Wounds

These are very serious wounds which penetrate into one of the body cavities, for example, the thorax or abdomen. The internal organs may be affected. This type of injury could be caused through a horse staking himself on a fence or becoming impaled on a sharp object. Initial first aid involves stemming serious bleeding and covering the opening with sterile gauze or bandage to prevent air being drawn into the cavity, which would lead to contamination.

A deep hole should be packed with sterile gauze and bandaged or taped in place. If the penetrating object is still present, do not try to remove it. Keep the horse still, cover the point of entry with a clean dressing and call the vet. The horse may need to be sedated to facilitate the safe removal of the object.

CONTUSED WOUNDS (BRUISING)

Bruising can occur as a result of a kick, fall or becoming cast. The force causes haemorrhage, oedema and inflammation, often without breaking the skin. Treatment involves immobilization and the application of cold treatments (hosing and ice packs). Once the initial pain has subsided, hot and cold fomentations can be applied to encourage the dispersal of accumulated fluids.

After 2–3 days, large haematomas may need to be drained. The vet may make a hole in the lowest part of the haematoma which will need to be kept open to allow complete drainage. The hole should be kept scrupulously clean to avoid contamination. The vet may prescribe anti-inflammatory drugs.

TENDON INJURIES

The flexor tendons of the forelimb are very prone to injury, particularly in performance horses. A common injury is **tendonitis** – straining and inflammation of the tendon fibres. The tendons of the lower limb are under varying degrees of pressure, depending upon whether the horse is simply walking around a field or competing. Whatever work the horse is doing, the tendons are constantly changing – the old, worn fibres being replaced by new, young ones.

THE NATURE OF TENDONS

Tendons are made up of bundles of collagen fibrils, known as **fascicles**, which are arranged longitudinally. Within the fascicles are the collagen-producing cells, known as **fibroblasts** (mentioned earlier when discussing wound healing).

Collagen is an inelastic fibrous protein, which makes up the bulk of all skin, connective tissue, bone, cartilage and tendons. The type of collagen of which tendons are formed has a crimped structure which, if stretched, pulls straight, so helping to absorb and reduce stress and strain. However, as the collagen fibrils become older and worn they lose their crimped effect, which results in a loss of elasticity.

The rate at which new collagen fibrils replace old is dependent upon the adequate flow of blood bringing nutrients and oxygen to the area, and also upon correct pH levels. Blood circulation is increased and improved by regular exercise, therefore the collagen fibres are replaced more quickly, resulting in stronger tendons. The horse in less demanding work will not have such strong tendons, and should never be over-exerted suddenly. Furthermore, repeated loading of a tendon tends to stabilize its mechanical response, making it both more elastic and stiffer. In this state it is less susceptible to damage. For this reason it is important to warm the horse up gradually at the beginning of exercise.

Under normal, healthy conditions the collagen in tendons should be renewed approximately every six months. However, interference with the oxygen supply, perhaps as a result of injury which impairs circulation, may lead to degenerative changes within the tendon, which will further complicate the healing process.

CAUSES OF TENDON INJURY

Conformation faults. Various faults of conformation may cause or contribute to tendon injury:
- Relative to the size of the horse, long cannon bones will have long tendons, which are more susceptible to strain than shorter tendons.

- Limbs which are too small in relation to the size of the body may not be strong enough to support it properly.
- Excessively sloping pastern/foot axes exert too much pressure on the tendons.

Degenerative injury. Poor circulation, and therefore poor oxygen supply, may be a result of faulty foot conformation. In such cases the collagen fibres are not replaced regularly as previously described, the existing collagen loses its elasticity and is unable to withstand any level of stress. If subjected to regular stress, warning signs of heat and swelling may appear.

Contracted tendons. As a result of contraction of the digital flexor tendons the heel may be raised and the fetlock joint straightened. In severe cases the front of the fetlock joint may even touch the ground. This condition, sometimes referred to as 'knocking over', may be present at birth, in which case it may cause problems with foaling. When the foal is standing on 'tiptoe' as a result of contracted tendons this is referred to as 'ballerina syndrome'. Alternatively, the condition may develop suddenly in youngsters as a result of tendon injury, infection or dietary deficiency.

Muscle fatigue. Fatigue may result from bad going or the over-exertion of an unfit horse. Once the parent muscle becomes fatigued it becomes less coordinated, placing extra strain on the tendon, which may then be overstretched.

Mechanical injury may result from the horse striking into himself whilst jumping or galloping. (Such injury may also be the result of misfortune, for example, putting a foot down a rabbit hole).

SIGNS AND EFFECTS OF TENDON INJURY

Early signs include localized heat and swelling – although the horse may not be lame initially. With more serious tendon strain, referred to as 'breaking down', there will be a greater degree of inflammation accompanied by severe lameness. The tendon may appear 'bowed' when viewed from the side.

Depending upon the nature and extent of the injury, the tendon fibres are torn or stretched. This may lead to haemorrhaging within the tendon, which stimulates other cell-bearing fluids to enter the injured site. These fluids seep through from adjacent tissues in order to clear away debris such as dead tissue and to fight against infection of the damaged area. However, as a result of cells dying, toxic substances are formed. These irritate the surrounding tissue and this further stimulates the flow of blood to the area, leading to inflammation.

Where inflammation occurs beneath an annular ligament, extreme pressure is exerted on the inflamed area. This usually reduces circulatory flow, which can then lead to tissue death and bowed tendons ('low bow').

After an injury, the limb is usually naturally immobilized (the horse is reluctant to move) – this is a result of the pain and swelling. Further immobi-lization is enforced as the horse has to rest. This lack of movement leads to impaired circulation, as venous return is dependent upon muscle contraction.

As a result of the impaired circulation, the area becomes engorged with blood, fluids and cells, which solidify to form a haematoma. In areas of intense inflammation, especially where a haematoma has formed, there is a danger of **adhesions** forming as a result of the loss of movement. Adhesions are areas where the healing tissues become stuck to over- and underlying tissues, which further limits movement. If adhesions are stretched, they break down and cause damage to adjacent areas.

In association with tendon fibre damage, or as reaction to an injury or blow, the tendon sheath may become inflamed. This is known as **tenosynovitis**.

ITQ 28 Why does the amount of exercise a horse has affect the strength of his tendons?

THE HEALING PROCESS

A few days after injury, new blood vessels begin to permeate the injured area, pushing their way through the engorged and swollen tissues. These blood vessels carry building cells for repair to the site, and also remove damaged tissue. The repair cells lay down collagen fibres to form a scar (granulation tissue).

The repair collagen is not arranged longitudinally, but is placed in random fashion, which reduces the strength of the tendon. Eventually the fibres realign and are replaced, although the collagen with which they are replaced is of a weaker type. After a year or so this may be replaced again, this time with a stronger type of collagen.

Whenever dealing with tendon injuries it is necessary to bear in mind the time taken before the tendons are remodelled – in the year following injury the tendons will not be at full strength.

TREATING TENDON INJURIES

To determine the severity of the injury, the vet will recommend that an accurate diagnosis be obtained through ultrasound scanning (see Chapter 3). This will assist in planning the best course of treatment.

Although inflammation heralds the healing process, the priority, for the reasons described above, is to immediately control and reduce it. Cold treatments/hydrotherapy and support bandaging should be used initially and the vet may prescribe an anti-inflammatory drug such as phenylbutazone (bute). Box rest will be essential in severe cases, to prevent the horse from using the limb and causing further damage.

It is thought that controlled passive motion with slight tension on the injured tendon, e.g. walking in hand, in the acute repair stage (granulation tissue deposition) helps with orientation of the fibrils and reduces adhesion formation.

However, finding a balance between mild tension to promote repair and more severe tension which compromises healing, remains a problem.

Tendon injuries should be monitored through ultrasound at three-month intervals. Once the initial repair period is complete (this can only be determined by ultrasound scanning) most horses are turned out for 9–18 months before resuming work and many never return to hard/fast work.

ITQ 29 State three conformational faults which may contribute to tendon injury.

1.

2.

3.

ITQ 30 Give an outline description of what happens when a tendon 'breaks down'.

ITQ 31 In terms of tendon injury healing, what are adhesions?

BONE FRACTURES

Bone fractures are classified as wounds because of the associated soft tissue trauma.

THE NATURE OF BONE

Bone may fracture if it is subjected to excessive trauma or stress. In order to understand why this may happen, and what happens during the healing process, it is necessary to know something of the processes of **remodelling** and **mineralization**.

Bone is a hard, supportive tissue, but it is far from inert. It continually changes its shape and mass through the process of remodelling and mineralization. The nutrients and oxygen needed for these processes are supplied to the bone by an extensive network of blood vessels. Bone acts as a store for calcium and phosphorus, the removal or deposition of which are affected by hormonal influences, nutrition and physical stresses on the bone.

As bone matures, along with the horse, it becomes **mineralized**, i.e. space that was occupied by cellular fluid is filled by the minerals, calcium and phosphorus. When the horse is fully mature the minerals make up 95% of the bone. Mineralization increases bone density and rigidity, making it more resistant to deforming forces. In addition, the cross-sectional area increases with skeletal maturity, resulting in strong bone. Also, bone increases or decreases in mass in response to stresses placed on it. The mechanical forces applied by consistent exercise lead to an increase in bone mass and mineralization as the bone gradually adapts to cope with an increasing workload. It is known that daily exercise consisting of short periods of vigorous work (following a warm-up period) promotes optimum bone strengthening. However, hard and fast work, especially without sufficient preparation, can lead to damage which, although microscopic, may culminate in a series of micro-cracks in the bone. The first part of the normal remodelling process in response to this involves the removal of damaged bone via the channels of the Haversian system (the central tunnels and layers of the bone). Healthy bone cells are then deposited, which repair the micro-cracks. This is known to take approximately five months. However, the initial stage of remodelling, when the damaged material is removed, actually causes further weakening of the bone. It is at this time that the horse is susceptible to stress fractures.

Of course, not all fractures are the result of stress (i.e. the overloading of a weakened bone); they can also occur as the result of trauma, e.g. a kick from another horse. Although all bones are susceptible to fracture, those most commonly affected in the horse are the long pasterns, cannon bones, pedal bones, sesamoids and splint bones.

A final point relating to the processes of modelling and mineralization is that the inactivity and reduced loading that are essential following a fracture lead to **demineralization** and the resorption of existing bone cells, and bone-forming cells become inactive. The cumulative result is weaker bone – this must be borne in mind when bringing a horse who has been on box rest back into work. *Rehabilitation must proceed slowly.*

ITQ 32 Name the process by which bone mass increases or decreases.

ITQ 33 List the three factors which affect the removal or deposition of minerals within bone.

1.
2.
3.

ITQ 34 What physiological changes occur within bone in response to consistent exercise?

ITQ 35 What type of exercise promotes optimum bone strength?

ITQ 36 What physiological changes occur within bone in response to inactivity and reduced loading?

ITQ 37 In terms of limb fracture, which bones are most commonly affected in the horse?

TYPES OF FRACTURE

Fractures are classified according to the type of break – this range of classifications is very extensive. To the layperson, the broad categories are more relevant, and it is these we shall discuss. Within these main categories we need to consider that a fracture may affect a small bone, e.g. tarsal, carpal bones, for which treatment is often possible, or a long limb bone, which is much more serious. Additionally fractures may be **open**, i.e. exposed, or **closed**, i.e. not exposed.

Simple fracture. This is the most common. The bone is broken clean across, and the break is described as transverse, longitudinal or oblique, according to its direction. There may be damage to surrounding tissue.

Compound fracture. Also known as an **open fracture**. The skin is damaged and the break is exposed. This is a very serious injury, which may be prone to heavy bleeding and infection.

Comminuted fracture. There is a lot of splintering, involving a number of pieces of bone.

Incomplete fracture. The bone breaks partly across but the **periosteum** (bone membrane) generally does not break. This is also known as a '**greenstick**' **fracture** and may occur in young foals whose bones are still immature.

Stress fracture. As mentioned earlier, fast work may lead to bone damage and the formation of micro-cracks; the first stage of remodelling weakens the bone further. The bone fractures as a result of excessive loading whilst in this weakened state. Many stress fractures do not show up on X-ray but can be detected through a bone scan. If the damage is limited then rest may be enough to facilitate healing. However, if the fracture is extensive it may not be possible to treat it.

SIGNS OF A FRACTURE

The horse will *usually* show one or a combination of the following signs:
- Loss of use of limb.
- Severe lameness.
- No weightbearing on limb.
- Deformity of limb.
- Unnatural mobility of limb. (If the pelvis is fractured the horse will be unable to walk properly – he may move with a sideways, crab-like movement.)
- Apparent shortening of length of limb.
- Pain and swelling.
- Crepitus – grating sound as bone endings move.
- Shock signs – pale mucous membranes; severe sweating; elevated heart and respiratory rates.

ITQ 38 List five types of fracture and give a brief description of each.

1.

2.

3.

4.

5.

ITQ 39 List four signs of a fracture.

1.
2.
3.
4.

PROGNOSIS FOLLOWING A FRACTURE

Developments in modern veterinary surgery including the use of rigid internal fixation, bone grafting techniques, improved anaesthetic procedures and better casting materials have generally improved the prognosis for a limb fracture. However, the outcome of any injury will depend upon the following factors:

- Which bone is fractured.
- The nature of the fracture.
- The nature of other associated injuries.
- The initial management of the fracture at the scene of the accident.
- The age and temperament of the horse.
- Finances, insurance cover and value of the horse.
- The usefulness of the horse upon recovery.

(The last two are not part of the clinical prognosis: they are practical factors that may have a bearing on whether treatment is carried out, rather than whether it might be successful.)

INITIAL FRACTURE MANAGEMENT

First aid measures must be taken at the scene of an accident to prevent further deterioration of the injury whilst waiting for the veterinary surgeon to arrive. The outcome of many fractures is determined by the success of this initial treatment.

The aims of first aid where a fracture is suspected are:

- To minimize further damage to the bone ends and surrounding soft tissue.
- To prevent bone from penetrating skin and the fracture becoming contaminated.
- To prevent further damage to nerves and blood vessels in the limb.
- To stabilize the limb, thus reducing the horse's anxiety.

The limb must be very well padded and supported to help minimize the effects of the injury and to reduce subsequent damage. Unless stabilized, closed fractures may become open and damaged soft tissue will be susceptible to infection and a localized loss of blood supply (**ischaemia**).

The horse tends to become anxious about the damaged limb, and the fact that he cannot control it. The anxiety (and pain) result in sweating and repeated attempts to position the limb.

If the fracture is open, antibiotic therapy must start immediately, although the prognosis is not good, especially if there is little tissue covering the bone, or the wound has been contaminated.

Protective splints must neutralize the damaging forces exerted by the normal muscle movement. The limb must be splinted in such a way as to immobilize the area of the fracture. In an emergency, when no specialized splints are available, PVC guttering or wooden tool handles may be used to provide stability. The cotton wool is wrapped around the limb and compressed with the gauze bandages. The elastic bandages are then applied and the splints strapped tightly to the outside. The splints should not extend beyond the padding.

The joint above and below the break should be immobilized. This is difficult if the fracture is above the knee or hock, because it is impossible to bandage the stifle or elbow satisfactorily. It is not wise to attempt to splint these joints as that could cause displacement of the fracture.

To make up the heavily padded splints that are required, several rolls of cotton wool or similar, several rolls of gauze bandages and at least ten elasticated bandages are needed. When applied correctly this is termed a **Robert Jones bandage**, which consists of several thin layers of padding, each of which is firmly compressed by the gauze bandage then an elasticated bandage.

This is continued until the bandage is three times the diameter of the leg and like a tube in shape.

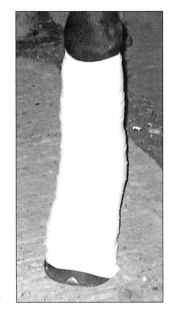

Figure 9 A Robert Jones bandage

The sound limb will also need a support bandage because it will be bearing much extra weight. If possible, the frog should also be supported in the sound limb – this can be achieved by taping a firm pad to the heel region of the foot. However, if the horse cannot bear weight on the injured limb this may not be possible.

A lot of pain will occur as a result of the bone ends moving – immobilization will help to alleviate this. (In addition to keeping the bone ends still, immobilization is crucial in that the blood supply for the healing process comes from the soft tissue and **endosteum** and, if this is not preserved, repair is compromised.) The endosteum is the layer of cells that line the medullary cavity (the hollow chamber within areas of compact bone).

The vet will administer analgesics, but will judge the level carefully as the horse must not be encouraged to use the limb.

Generally, the use of sedatives is avoided because of their effect on the cardiovascular system. A horse suffering from shock and haemorrhage will react adversely to any lowering of arterial blood pressure. Also, sedatives may lead to incoordination, which could result in further injury, especially during transit. However, in some circumstances a sedative has to be administered to prevent the horse from inflicting further damage, or to facilitate removal from the site of the accident. In such cases a short-acting agent such as xylazine may be administered intravenously by the vet.

> ITQ 40 Give three reasons why it is essential to immobilize a fracture as soon as possible after the accident.
>
> 1.
> 2.
> 3.

> ITQ 41 Describe briefly how a Robert Jones bandage is constructed.

When considering limb fracture, the limbs are divided into four functional segments, relating to both forelimbs and hind limbs.

Fractures of the Distal Forelimb (Forelimb Level 1)

This includes fractures of the long pastern bone, short pastern bone, sesamoid bones and the distal cannon bone. When a fracture occurs in this region it is likely to bend at the site of fracture as opposed to the fetlock joint, which it would do in the normal healthy state.

The leg should be supported above the knee, allowing the leg to hang with the toe pointing downward. Several light layers of cotton wool should be applied from

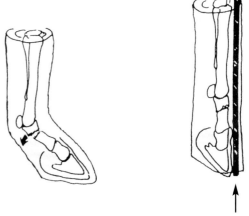

Splinting to prevent bending at the fetlock joint and fracture site

Figure 10 Fracture of the distal forelimb

just below the knee to the ground. A splint of wood or plastic guttering should be applied on the dorsal aspect and taped firmly in position to prevent bending. Padding must be applied at the top of the splint to prevent rubbing.

Fractures of the Mid-distal Forelimb (Forelimb Level 2)

These include fractures of the mid-shaft and proximal metacarpus (cannon bone) and distal radius.

It will be necessary to splint the whole limb, applying a Robert Jones bandage from the ground to the elbow.

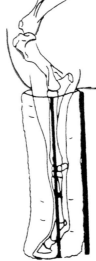

Figure 11 Fracture of the mid-distal forelimb

Fractures of the Mid-proximal Forelimb (Forelimb Level 3)

These include fractures of the shaft and proximal aspect of the radius. Because of the musculature of the leg, when a fracture occurs in this region it will cause the limb to abduct (move away from the body). Abduction will cause damage to the skin, resulting in an open fracture.

Splinting must prevent abduction and stabilize the fracture site. A Robert Jones bandage is applied, encasing the whole limb, and a lateral splint is applied from the ground to mid-scapula. Padding is necessary where the splint lies over the scapula and rib cage.

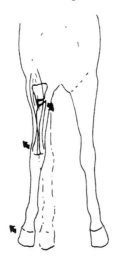 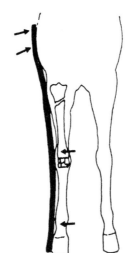

Figure 12 Fracture of the mid-proximal forelimb

Fractures of the High Forelimb (Forelimb Level 4)

This includes any structure proximal to the elbow joint, e.g. the humerus, ulna or scapula. Fractures of these bones are well protected by muscles in the area, which reduces the need for stabilization. However, the horse will not be able to fix his elbow or knee – both will appear to have 'dropped', making it impossible for the horse to bear any weight.

Splinting for this type of fracture involves extending the knee, applying padding and taping a splint caudally to the knee.

Fractures of the Distal Hind Limb (Hind Limb Level 1)

These affect the same bones as in Forelimb Level 1 and are treated in the same way. When applying the Robert Jones bandage, the limb should be held above the hock and extended. It may be necessary to sedate the horse to prevent him from withdrawing the limb.

Fractures of the Mid-distal Hind Limb (Hind Limb Level 2)

This region extends from the distal cannon to proximal cannon. Fractures should be splinted by taping a lateral and caudal splint on a Robert Jones bandage from the foot to the top of the os calcis.

Fractures of the Mid-proximal Hind Limb (Hind Limb Level 3)

This region includes the hock and tibia. A fracture in this area causes disruption of the simultaneous extension and flexion of hock and stifle joints. This means that flexion of the stifle will no longer result in flexion of the hock, but causes the fracture site to move – resulting in trauma.

Also, because of the musculature in the hind limb, abduction will occur. A Robert Jones bandage should be applied from the ground as high proximally as possible. A splint should be applied laterally, using either a bent metal bar or a long, straight piece of wood.

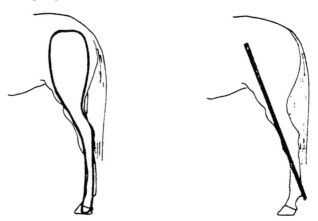

Figure 13 Fracture of the mid-proximal hind limb

Fractures of the Femur (Hind Limb Level 4)

It is not possible to splint the femur, but the large muscle mass in the area will help to stabilize the fracture site.

TRANSPORTING THE INJURED HORSE

Once the temporary stabilization of the limb is complete and all other first aid measures have been attended to, the horse can be moved to the veterinary hospital. An ambulance trailer with a low, flat ramp should come to the horse.

Alternatively, a lorry may be used if the ramp is not too steep, a loading ramp is available or the horse is able to walk up the ramp.

Horses will often panic when trying to move with a splint applied – additional support should be given with people at the head and tail to aid stability. If possible, foals should be carried. Panic and the flight instinct can lead to a considerable worsening of the fracture in foals.

A horse with a forelimb injury should be loaded facing backwards where possible, to prevent excessive pressure being exerted on the limb when the lorry slows down.

For the same reason, a horse with a hind limb injury should face forwards. In a sideways-partitioned lorry the same rules apply to the left and right side legs as opposed to the fore and hind legs.

During transport, the horse should be confined with chest and rump bars and partitions. Ideally, he should be supported with a sling; if none is available, it may be necessary to improvise with straw bales. However, he should not be tied too tightly – he needs to move his head and neck to help keep his balance. An attendant must always travel with a foal to try to control his movements.

The vehicle must be driven with great care, avoiding sharp acceleration or braking. A haynet can be provided to try to distract the horse from his discomfort. The vet may administer xylazine, a short-acting tranquillizer which provides good analgesia for musculoskeletal pain.

Once the horse is at the veterinary hospital, the veterinary team will assess the horse's cardiovascular status and the state of hydration. A blood sample, assessment of the colouration of mucous membranes and capillary refill time will allow the vet to determine the level of dehydration. Fluid can be administered intravenously if needed.

The course of action to be taken will be decided upon after the injured limb has been X-rayed.

ITQ 42 List four important points to be considered when transporting a horse with a suspected limb fracture.

1.

2.

3.

4.

GENERAL CONSIDERATIONS IN FRACTURE TREATMENT

The main aim is to restore full use of the damaged limb as soon as possible. Prolonged immobilization will lead to various problems including joint stiffness, muscle atrophy, impaired circulation and soft tissue adhesions.

There will also be a risk of poor bony healing resulting in a 'malunion' of the broken limb and excessive callus formation.

Fractures in foals tend to repair more successfully than in the adult horse because foals are smaller and therefore their bones bear less weight. Also, the bone-producing cells are still very active, which promotes faster healing.

With an injury as serious as a limb fracture, the owner will be advised by the veterinary surgeon and team as to the daily progress and care of the horse.

FRACTURE HEALING

The healing of a fracture involves a complex sequence of changes; a number of different stages which overlap.

1. **Haemorrhage**. Bleeding occurs at the site of fracture as a result of the rupture of blood vessels in the periosteum, bone marrow and adjacent tissues. A large number of white blood cells will converge at the area.

2. **Haematoma formation**. The haemorrhage coagulates and envelopes the bone endings. The fragments of bone and connective tissue degenerate and are removed by phagocytes (white blood cells which adhere to and destroy invading bacteria). The haematoma then undergoes organization and is replaced by granulation tissue, forming a fibrous callus with non-aligned collagen fibres.

3. **Fibrous callus**. Fibroblasts (collagen-forming cells) produce many collagen fibres, which mainly lie parallel to the long axis of the bone. The callus anchors and seals the break by surrounding it. Tissue between the bone endings unites the break and further callus encircles it – this is known as **bridging**.

4. **Ossification**. The fibrous tissue is transformed into 'woven' bone by osteoblasts (bone-forming cells) forming a thick ring of new bone referred to as **hard callus**. The bone first produced is immature (spongy) and is later replaced by adult (lamellar) bone. When union is complete the thick ring of bone is remodelled. If the break does not heal well the new ring of bone will remain to provide strength.

CHAPTER SUMMARY

Despite excellent management practices horses generally have a great capacity to injure themselves. Sometimes these injuries can be very serious. This chapter has attempted to explain some of the types of injury which may occur and how they heal. It has not been written in an attempt to replace expert veterinary knowledge and advice, rather more as an aid for you, the horse owner/yard manager.

CHAPTER 3

CONTROLLING INFLAMMATION

The aims and objectives of this chapter are to explain:

- Methods of reducing and controlling inflammation.
- The benefits of each method.
- The types of therapy machine available
- The benefits of massage and support.
- The use of anti-inflammatory drugs.

The information given in this chapter must not be considered as a substitute for the advice of a veterinary surgeon. Advice must always be sought promptly for diagnostic and therapeutic purposes in the case of injury and/or lameness – delay may lead to irreparable damage and permanent unsoundness. The choice of treatment post-injury will depend upon the nature of the injury.

Methods of controlling inflammation include:
- Cryotherapy.
- Hydrotherapy.
- Heat therapy.
- Therapy machines which facilitate treatments such as magnetic field therapy, ultrasound and laser.
- Massage.
- Support.
- Anti-inflammatory drugs.

CRYOTHERAPY (COLD TREATMENTS)

Cryotherapy is the use of cooling as a means of treating injuries. The affected structures are cooled when heat is conducted to a cooler substance (e.g. water or ice) that has been applied to the skin. Cryotherapy is beneficial in the treatment of musculoskeletal trauma and pain caused by muscle spasm.

CONTRA-INDICATIONS

— Hypersensitivity to cold. Normal tissue can be damaged and pain caused rather than reduced.
— Impaired sensory function. Tissue cooling occurs more rapidly which

increases the risk and onset of tissue damage.
— Compromised circulation. Cold treatments may exacerbate defective circulation.

EFFECTS

The effects on the injured tissues include:

Hypometabolism. At a cellular level the metabolic response of the cells is reduced, thereby reducing their oxygen requirement, which decreases the risk of hypoxic damage (damage caused as a result of lack of oxygen).

Vasoconstriction. The blood vessels tighten and blood flow is reduced. This helps to control the formation of haematomas (blood-filled swellings) and oedema (fluid accumulation in tissues) beneath the skin. Vasoconstriction also helps stop bleeding in an open wound.

Vasodilation. This has been found to occur in the deep tissues of the area in response to the intense cold when ice treatments are in place for 10 minutes or more. Vasodilation follows vasoconstriction, and has the effect of increasing circulatory flow through the area.

Anti-inflammatory effects. In addition to inhibiting the release of histamines and neutrophils, cold reduces the damaging effects of collegenases (fibre-degrading enzymes). Cold therapy decreases the permeability of blood vessel walls, which reduces the amount of fluid that accumulates at the site of the wound.

Analgesia. As inflammation is reduced, so pain is eased. Cold treatments provide topical analgesia by interfering with nerve conduction, thereby slightly numbing the area.

Easing of muscle spasm. As pain is reduced, so muscle spasm begins to ease. Muscles go into spasm in reaction to pain – the tightness of this spasm further heightens the pain and interferes with the circulatory flow which, in turn, reduces the oxygen supply to the area. Any interference with the supply of oxygen may lead to degenerative changes and tissue death (necrosis).

MODES OF APPLICATION

Cold treatments should start as soon as possible after injury to maximize its effect, and should be repeated every 4–6 hours within the first day.

Ice and Pressure

Used correctly, ice treatments can play a valuable role in reducing inflammation, but they should be applied with due care. Traditional ice treatments cause vasoconstriction of the superficial blood vessels, and prolonged exposure to intense cold causes neural and cellular damage, or 'ice burn'. If applied excessively, the reduction in blood flow can cause ischaemia (tissue death as a result of reduced blood flow). Because of the risk of tissue damage, ice treatments must not be placed in direct contact with the skin – a layer of damp cloth should be placed between the ice pack and the skin. (Dry cloth does not transmit cold so effectively.) Also, they must never be in position for longer than 30 minutes on any one area. Depending on modality, the optimum duration of treatment is 10–30 minutes.

Generally, the effectiveness of cold treatments is enhanced when they are combined with compression. However, once again, care must be taken – the pressure must be even and not excessive. Do not bandage too tightly over an ice pack. To prevent swelling, compression should be used between treatments; start bandaging at the distal (lower) end of the limb and work upwards for maximum effect.

During treatments, check skin temperature using a thermometer. Studies have shown the core temperature of the tissues should not drop below 15 °C.

Common forms of ice therapy include:

Ice massage. This is the simplest form. If the site of the injury permits, a block of ice can be rubbed over the injured area for 5–10 minutes. Ice blocks can be made by filling polystyrene cups with water and freezing. To use, peel half the cup away from the block, holding the remaining half. Use a slow, circular motion to massage the area. In this case, the massaging motion and duration of treatment make tissue damage unlikely.

Home-made cold dressings. Gamgee may be soaked in water and frozen in the deep freeze. This can then be bandaged in position. The ice particles begin to melt once the dressing is in place. Another useful form of cold poultice is kaolin spread between two sheets of polythene and then frozen. This makes an economical, reusable cold dressing.

Commercially produced cold dressings. There are various specialist preparations available on the market. These include gel-filled sachets and gel-impregnated bandages which, once frozen, remain cold for up to 3 hours. These preparations are designed to reach a therapeutic temperature level, so they may be used safely without the risk of tissue death.

Ice packs. These can be made at home, or purchased and kept in the freezer, ready for use. Whichever method is used, it is a good idea to keep several ice treatments ready-frozen.

To make an ice pack, fill a double-layered zip-locking freezer bag with two parts water and one part isopropyl alcohol, well mixed, and place in the freezer. The alcohol stops the pack from freezing into a solid block, making it easier to mould around the injured area. Another, more basic, form of ice pack can be made by filling a zip-locking bag with crushed ice and water.

When using commercial ice packs, follow the manufacturers' instructions. Homemade ice packs should be applied over a damp cloth or tube-grip bandage to prevent tissue damage. Periodically soak the cloth or tube-grip. As the ice pack warms, which can happen quickly if the limb is very inflamed, it will lose its effectiveness. Ice packs should be left in place for approximately 10–15 minutes.

Cold Hosing

The most common practice, cold hosing, should be carried out for at least 20 minutes at least three times daily, more if possible. Short periods of hosing are not of great benefit as the blood vessels do not have time to respond fully.

The heels must be plugged with petroleum jelly or a similar product and carefully dried after hosing to prevent cracking.

While traditional hosing is time-consuming, it is now possible to buy specially designed 'hose boots', often called 'aqua' or 'whirlpool' boots. These compress the water jet from the hose, giving a Jacuzzi-type massage which reduces oedema and improves circulation. Once the horse is accustomed to the boots he can be left standing tied up, which saves time spent holding the hosepipe, but he should not be left unattended in case there is a problem. However, great care is still needed with this method as the sole and frog quickly become soaked and the horn softens excessively. Iodine-based medications help to prevent this.

Other drawbacks to hosing (with or without boots) are that, as the water temperature is not controlled, it may not be cold enough to cool the deeper structures effectively. Also, in order to preserve water supplies, the use of hosepipes is banned in some areas of England during the summer.

Tubbing

This method involves encouraging the horse to stand with the affected limb immersed in a tub of crushed ice and water. As with hosing, precautions need to be taken to prevent cracked heels and the horse must stand still or the tub will be knocked over. The tub used should be of a type which will not split or tip over too easily. Garden centres sell a range of rubber trugs which can be adapted for this use. The ideal water temperature is around 16–18 °C – add more ice as necessary and agitate the water to ensure even temperature distribution.

Sea Water

The sea provides an excellent natural hydrotherapy treatment. The horse can either stand in or walk through the sea. (Obviously this will only be of use to those who live near a coastline.)

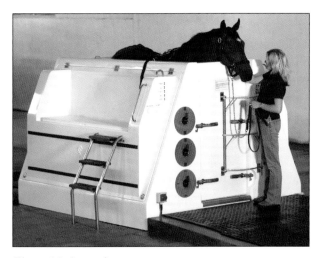

Figure 14 An equine spa

Therapeutic Spas

Equine 'walk-in' spas are increasing in popularity and use. The water temperature is maintained between 2 and 4 °C to minimize inflammation. Salt is added to the water and the solution acts as a hypertonic poultice with a natural healing effect. Increased salt concentration increases pressure which further aids the dispersal of fluid. At present it is mainly equine therapy and rehabilitation yards which offer such facilities, although some racehorse trainers now have spas installed on their yards.

HEAT THERAPY
CONTRA-INDICATIONS

Do not use heat therapy:

- If severe infection of the deeper tissues is suspected, since vasodilation can cause the spread of toxins. However, the localized application of heat (as in poulticing and hot-tubbing) can be useful in drawing out exudate resulting from local, relatively mild, infection.

- In advance of other therapies (such as the administration of antibiotics) which may act to treat, and thus reduce, the infection.

- In the acute stages of inflammation. Cold is more effective in the acute stage.

- If skin irritation exists, as heat may exacerbate the condition.

EFFECTS

The effects on the injured tissues include:

Analgesia. The sensation of pain is decreased.

Hypermetabolism. At a cellular level, the cells' metabolic activity is increased – which, in turn, increases blood flow.

Increased blood flow. Circulation is enhanced, improving oxygen supply and toxin removal. This promotes healing.

Relief of muscle spasm and improvement in the elasticity of scar tissue, which increases the range of movement. Heat therapy is an effective precursor to stretching exercises.

> ITQ 43 Why should heat therapy not be used to reduce inflammation if infection is present in the deeper tissues?

MODES OF APPLICATION
Hot Packs

Commercially prepared hot packs are available. These can be heated in the microwave as per the instructions prior to application. Alternatively, a hot-water bottle can be filled with hot water and held in position. Use a layer of towelling or similar between the heat source and the skin to prevent tissue damage and burning.

Poultices

As mentioned in Chapter 2, poultices help to relieve bruising, clean wounds, draw out infection and reduce inflammation. To prevent burning, always ensure that poultices are not too hot when applied; test the temperature on the back of your hand. Common types of poultice include Animalintex, a ready-prepared lint dressing which is cut to size and soaked in very hot water. Wring out the excess water, apply to the injury and cover with polythene. Either bandage into position using Gamgee as padding or, if using on an area where bandaging is impractical, hold in place with waterproof sticking plaster. (Animalintex may also be used as a cold dressing.)

Hot Tubbing

This is a form of treatment to ease bruising of the lower leg, draw out infection and clean puncture wounds. Use a strong rubber bucket full of hot (but not too hot) water with approximately 50 g Epsom salts in solution. Rub petroleum jelly onto the horse's heels to prevent cracking, pick out and scrub the foot, then immerse the injured limb. The horse must be encouraged to stand still with his foot in the bucket. Add hot water regularly and keep the foot immersed for 20 minutes. Repeat at least twice daily.

Fomentation

Hot and cold fomentations can be used to help reduce swelling. To do this you need a bucket of very cold water, two small hand towels and a bucket of very hot water. Keep the kettle hot so that you can top up the hot water. Soak each towel and wring out the cold one. Hold this over the bruise for a minute or two, then wring out the very hot towel and hold that over the bruise.

Repeating the alternate hot and cold applications will stimulate the circulation by causing the blood vessels to dilate then constrict. The blood and fluid which have gathered beneath the skin should start to disperse. You will need to do this for at least 20 minutes three times a day until the bruising has eased.

Infrared Radiation

Infrared (IR) radiation is electromagnetic radiation which, when absorbed by the body, has a heating effect. Solariums consist of lamps which emit short-wave infrared radiation. IR can be used to ease muscle stiffness and prior to mobilization exercises.

Short-wave Diathermy

The deep tissues of the body (including bone) can be warmed by means of a machine emitting a high-frequency alternating current. Because damage can easily occur through overheating of the deep tissues, this machine must only be used by a qualified person. It should never be carried out if bone screws or metalware are in place.

(Although this therapy is mechanically based, it has been included here because it is specifically a heat therapy, whereas those therapies discussed in the next section, while they may include a heating role, are more complex in their functioning and effects.)

THERAPY MACHINES

A wide range of specialist therapies are now available for the treatment of wounds and inflammation. These therapies are in use by physiotherapists and other expert personnel at clinics and rehabilitation centres. Many of the machines are available to purchase, but it must be stressed that they should be used in accordance with the veterinary surgeon's or physiotherapist's advice and only by a trained person.

MAGNETIC FIELD THERAPY

Much research has gone into the effects of pulsating and static magnetic field therapy in the treatment of both hard (bone) and soft (muscle and tendon) tissue damage. Certain pulses of magnetic field energy increase cell activity and improve circulation, which promotes the healing process. Research suggests that different pulses affect different tissues.

Static magnetic therapy is administered through the use of strategically placed magnets which remain in place almost continuously. There is a wide range of magnetic therapy boots, rugs and straps available which are claimed to promote healing and ease arthritis.

Pulsating magnetic (electromagnetic) therapy may be administered through a mains or battery operated unit via a rug or, if treating a leg injury, a boot.

The manufacturers give full treatment instructions which, together with the advice of an expert, should be followed carefully.

ULTRASOUND

Sound may be defined as vibrating waves travelling through a medium such as air. The length, velocity and frequency of sound waves are measured in **cycles per second**, which are expressed as **hertz**. A **kilohertz** (KHz) is 1,000 cycles per second; a **megahertz** (MHz) is 1 million cycles per second. The normal limit of human hearing is around 20 KHz – ultrasound waves cannot be perceived by the human ear as they have a frequency well above this.

Ultrasonic waves are, in fact, reflected by air; it causes them to bounce back upon themselves. However, when emitted from an ultrasound machine used by a trained person, ultrasonic waves may be used for scanning tissue for measurement, diagnosis and treatment.

When used as treatment, ultrasound waves are converted to heat in the tissues. The treatment is best used for deep heat penetration of muscles, and for nerve damage, tendon injury, bursitis and scars. Through the treatment, blood flow is increased, helping to reduce inflammation and muscle spasm, and scar tissue may become more elastic after ultrasound treatment.

Ultrasound is not of value in cases of bone damage, and can actually damage bone. For this reason, it should not be used over the spine. Furthermore, it should not be used in acute injuries (as it may cause haematoma formation) or over metal implants or recent surgical sites.

Also, if ultrasound is used for too long, at too high a temperature, by an inexperienced person, damage may occur within the deep structures.

Ultrasound Machines

These machines, originally designed for human usage, may have three frequency settings; 0.75 MHz, 1 MHz and 3 MHz. However, the most commonly used machines often have only the I MHz setting, which makes them less controllable when treating structures of differing depths.

The machines are mains operated, the generator being within an earthed metal box, on which are the control dials. The dials control the setting of timing, intensity (ultrasonic waves are measured as watts/cm^2) and whether the waves are pulsed or continuous.

Attached to the generator by a lead is the transducer, or treatment head. Attached to the metal plate of the transducer is a special type of crystal (usually quartz or barium titanate,) which is capable of vibrating according to the setting of the machine (thus, at 1 MHz the crystal must vibrate at 1 million cycles per second).

The high-frequency current is transmitted from the crystal to the metal plate, which produces an ultrasonic wave. This wave has to pass through a medium other than air – a special coupling gel may be used or, in treating a limb, the affected area may be immersed in water.

When used for diagnostic purposes, the emitter and receiver are in a probe. Depending upon the depth of penetration needed, a setting of 3, 5 or 7.5 MHz is used.

Method of Treatment

The area to be treated is clipped closely. If the **immersion method** is being used, the affected limb is submerged in a strong tub of water. All air bubbles must be rubbed out of the hair, so that the ultrasound waves are not reflected back. The treatment head is held parallel to the limb approximately 1–2 cm away and moved in a slow circular or parallel motion. This head should always be kept in motion to avoid overheating the tissue.

If the **contact method** is to be used, the treatment surface of the transducer and the area to be treated should be well covered in the coupling gel. The transducer is placed firmly onto the area to be treated and the machine timing and intensity are set. With the contact method of treatment, the transducer head is moved in the same way as with the immersion method. As the beam travels through the coupling medium and the tissues of the body, its intensity is reduced. The effect of this is calculated and taken into account when treating the deeper structures. The lower the wattage per cm^2, the better. *Damage may occur if the treatment sessions are continued over too long a period.*

ITQ 44

a. What is ultrasound?

b. State three conditions which would benefit from the use of ultrasound:
1.
2.
3.

c. When used for therapeutic purposes, what effect does ultrasound have on the damaged tissue?

LASER

The word laser is an acronym: Light Amplification by Stimulated Emission of Radiation. Laser apparatus emits a beam of intense light which may be used for surgical, healing and/or analgesic purposes dependent upon the type of laser used.

- **High power** or **hot lasers** actually destroy tissue through intense heat and have been used in various forms of surgery with success.

- **Low power** or **cold lasers** do not destroy tissue, but have great therapeutic values.

When treatment is being given with a low power laser, the laser beam may be emitted in a pulsed or continuous wave; a pulsed beam is effective for analgesic purposes, while a continuous beam is generally used for healing.

Laser has an analgesic effect when used correctly on the acupuncture points. This treatment must be carried out approximately once a week by a trained person familiar with the many acupuncture points.

If a continuous beam is used on an open wound, it penetrates the tissues and is absorbed by the cells, where it acts as an extra energy source. This extra energy accelerates the healing process by helping collagen to be produced more rapidly. It also has an antibacterial effect and so reduces the incidence of infection.

Laser has been used to treat superficial joint and bone injuries, tendon and ligament conditions and old fibrous scar tissue. This treatment reduces the time taken to recover quite noticeably, even though there is no sensation felt by the horse while the beam is penetrating the damaged tissues.

If the treatment starts within 24 hours of the injury occurring, the formation of proud flesh can be completely prevented. This leads to minimal scarring and normal coat re-growth.

Laser is generally effective to a depth of 10–15 mm, the depth of penetration and the effectiveness of the beam being dependent on the wavelength and frequency of the emitted beam.

The apparatus should only be used by a trained and skilled operator as, used incorrectly, laser may have adverse effects on the injured site. Because of the risk of eye damage, it is important not to look directly at the laser source. There is still much research being carried out in the field of laser therapy.

> **ITQ 45 How does laser treatment assist in wound healing?**

MASSAGE AND SUPPORT

Used in conjunction with other forms of treatment to reduce inflammation, massage can have highly therapeutic qualities. It improves the local circulation, resulting in an increase in the rate at which waste products are removed from the area. There are two main types of massage.

Friction massage. When massaging the limbs, in particular the tendons, most benefit is gained from small movements concentrated in one area – the fingers press, following the line of the tissues beneath the skin. A lubricant should be used to allow the fingers to slide over the coat easily.

Mechanical massage machines. These may be hand-held units or specialized adhesive pads. The affected area of the limb should be fitted with a tube-grip stocking and the machine worked over this to prevent a skin reaction. The horse should initially be allowed to become used to a low level of vibration, which can be increased gradually.

Treatment by either form of massage will probably be necessary three times daily, for 30 minutes per session, continued until the condition has noticeably improved.

Support is an important aid in preventing excessive inflammation of an area. In extreme cases, the vet may apply a plaster cast. After cold treatments have been administered, support bandages should be used to prevent a sudden surge of blood and fluids back to the area. The method of bandaging for support has been described in Chapter 2.

ANTI-INFLAMMATORY DRUGS

When an area of tissue becomes damaged, a chemical known as **arachidonic acid** is released. This is then acted upon by the enzyme **cyclo-oxygenase**. The result of this interaction is the conversion of arachidonic acid into **prostaglandins**, the chemicals which cause the symptoms of heat, pain and swelling and also increase the sensitivity of pain receptors in the area.

Anti-inflammatory drugs which may be administered to reduce these painful effects of inflammation can be divided into two main groups: corticosteroids and non-steroidal anti-inflammatories (NSAIDs).

CORTICOSTEROIDS

Cortisol, a natural compound, was originally used in anti-inflammatory corticosteroids, but it is now more common for synthetic corticosteroids to be used. The exact manner in which these drugs act on inflammation is not definitely known, but it is considered that they act within the nuclei of the affected cells, causing an alteration to the production of proteins.

Their anti-inflammatory effects include:

- Stabilization of cell membranes (reducing the release of damaging enzymes).
- Inhibiting prostaglandin release.
- Inhibiting white blood cell migration.
- Reducing fibrosis – fibrin deposition.
- Reducing fluid accumulation.

However, since they inhibit the actual healing process and suppress the immune response, they should not be used in open wounds or in the presence of infection.

Corticosteroids may be injected directly into the inflamed area (for example, into a joint) or administered intravenously. Generally, a single dose can be given without serious side-effects, but prolonged treatment can be dangerous.

> ### ITQ 46
>
> a. Name the chemical that is released when an area of tissue is damaged.
>
> b. This chemical is acted upon by the enzyme cyclo-oxygenase. What chemical is produced as a result and what effect does it have?

NON-STEROIDAL ANTI-INFLAMMATORY DRUGS (NSAIDS)

These drugs are chemically unrelated to cortisol, being of a different chemical structure.

The non-steroidal drugs in use include the well-known **phenylbutazone** (**bute**) and the less well-known **meclofenamic acid, flunixin meglumine** and **naproxen**. These drugs act by neutralizing the enzyme cyclo-oxygenase –

without this chemical catalyst the arachidonic acid cannot be converted into prostaglandins, so the signs of inflammation will subside.

All drugs should be administered under veterinary advice as all have side-effects and the random use of them, particularly if given in too large a dosage, can have serious long-term effects.

TOPICAL ANTI-INFLAMMATORY PREPARATIONS

Gels containing salicylate, e.g. Tensolvet, are topical anti-inflammatories with analgesic properties. Tensolvet increases the blood flow through the underlying skin and promotes the early resorption of haematoma and oedematous swelling. Impervious gloves should be worn when applying such gels to prevent absorption through the skin. The gel is applied up to four times a day – the manufacturer's directions must be followed.

ITQ 47 Why should corticosteroids not be used when infection is present or the wound is open?

ITQ 48 Name two non-steroidal anti-inflammatory drugs in common use.

1.

2.

BLISTERING AND FIRING

These so-called 'therapies' have become less common today and are not advocated by the veterinary profession in the UK.

Blistering involves the application of an irritant substance such as mercuric iodide, which causes inflammation and blistering. The outdated and unproven reasons for doing this are that circulation will be improved to bring about healing, thus benefiting the damaged tendons, and that the resultant scar tissue will provide a strengthened support to the area.

Firing is supposed to produce the same results – the skin being pierced either in parallel lines (line firing) or in a matrix of dots (pin firing), by a red-hot iron. Research has proved that blistering and firing do not enhance the healing process but actually hinder it and cause unnecessary suffering to the horse.

CHAPTER SUMMARY

If inflammation is not controlled and reduced, healing will be compromised. This increases the risk of further complications such as adhesions occurring and, when inflammation is present, the horse will be in great pain so, for humane reasons, steps must be taken to reduce inflammation.

Many of the treatments are very simple and effective, but new developments and advances in technology mean there is an increasing range of sophisticated items of equipment now available.

It is essential that operators of therapy machines are trained in their use as more harm than good can be done if they are used incorrectly. Most importantly, veterinary advice must be sought and followed.

CHAPTER 4

INFECTIOUS DISEASES

The aims and objectives of this chapter are to explain the signs, causes and treatment of:

- Viral and bacterial diseases of the respiratory tract.
- General viral infections.
- General bacterial diseases.
- Toxins from other sources – poisoning.

RESPIRATORY DISEASES – GENERAL SIGNS

Before discussing specific viral and bacterial respiratory diseases, we will look at some common signs of respiratory disease, and what causes them. The common signs are:

Excess mucus production. The airways are lined with mucous membranes, the secretions of which help to trap dust particles or bacteria. Hair-like cilia 'sweep' these particles to the throat, from where they are swallowed. They are later excreted via the digestive tract.

As a result of excessive debris and/or the invasion of bacteria, the mucus becomes thicker and stickier. It is then far more difficult for the horse to shift, with the result that the bronchioles become blocked. This reduces the capacity for gaseous exchange, so the horse is unable to breathe and work efficiently. The cilia are damaged and unable to function properly.

Coughing. The cough is triggered by irritation of the airways and helps to shift the sticky mucus. If the ailment is infectious, the coughing process leads to widespread dispersal of infectious bacteria or viruses.

Restriction of airways. The muscular walls of the airways contract in response to irritation from dust particles, bacteria, etc. When disease is present, the muscles becomes very sensitive and over-constricted. This condition, which restricts the free passage of air, is known as **bronchospasm**. Air passing through the much-restricted airways will rush through more quickly, causing a wheezing noise.

Inflammation. The excessive irritation leads to a sensitive, inflamed state of the lining of the airways. This inflammation causes narrowing of the airways, which again restricts airflow.

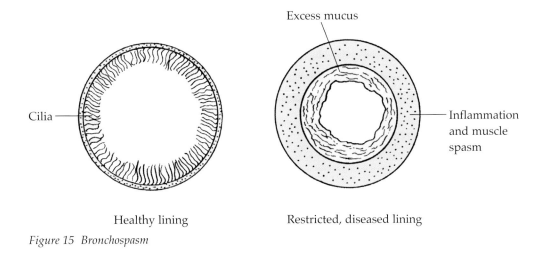

Excess mucus

Cilia

Inflammation
and muscle
spasm

Healthy lining

Restricted, diseased lining

Figure 15 Bronchospasm

VIRAL INFECTIONS OF THE RESPIRATORY TRACT
EQUINE INFLUENZA

The international transportation of horses has become more practical and affordable, particularly for those involved in competition, racing and sales. However, with the equine population travelling greater distances both at home and abroad, the risk of spreading infectious diseases increases.

Causes

Equine influenza is a highly infectious disease of the lower respiratory tract, caused by a group of myxoviruses. The two main types are **A/Equi 1** (first isolated in Prague in 1956, then Cambridge 1963) and **A/Equi 2** (Miami 1963). The latter type is particularly harmful, killing foals and yearlings and causing permanent lung damage in older horses. Since these two strains of virus produce different antigens, they can be identified separately. More recent A/Equi 2 strains are Fontainbleu (1979), Brentwood (1979), Kentucky (1981), Suffolk (1989), Borlange (1991) and Newmarket (1993).

Signs

The strain of the virus influences the range of signs shown, but some of the following will be evident.
- General lethargy, dullness and loss of appetite.
- Fever – a sharp rise in temperature, up to 39–41 °C (103–106 °F) which lasts 1–4 days, reducing as the condition progresses.
- Harsh, dry cough at rest and exercise (prior to diagnosis), lasting 2–3 weeks, or even longer.
- Nasal discharge that is initially clear and watery, but becomes thicker and pus-like as the disease progresses.
- Mucous membranes of the eyes and nostrils may be inflamed.
- Difficulty in breathing.
- There may be difficulty in swallowing and swollen glands (submandibular lymph nodes).

Equine influenza spreads rapidly through a yard as each cough expels large quantities of infective virus into the air, which is then inhaled by other horses. The incubation period is short, ranging from 1–3 days – the horse may begin to show signs as early as 24 hours after initial infection. The horse remains infectious for 6–10 days after the onset of signs.

Treatment

Call the vet, who may administer antibiotics to prevent secondary bacterial infection. The vet may also send a nasopharyngeal swab of discharge and/or a blood sample to the laboratory for analysis to determine the exact strain of virus or to check whether the signs are a result of infection by the equine herpes virus (EHV 1) – see later this chapter.

Adhere to all rules of isolation and sick nursing. Stringent precautions must be taken to ensure good stable hygiene.

Ensure a dust-free environment and very good ventilation.

After an attack, a long period of rest is essential; mildly affected animals may recover in 2–3 weeks, but those severely affected may need as long as 6 months to convalesce. It is extremely important that horses are not put back into work until they have completely recovered. As a general rule, for every day that the horse's temperature is raised above normal – 100.5 °F (38 °C) – he will need one week of complete rest.

There is always a risk of secondary conditions such as emphysema, chronic bronchitis and bacterial pneumonia occurring. Impaired circulation and jaundice may result if the horse returns to work too soon. Because the influenza virus also damages heart muscle and liver tissue, the repercussions could be permanent.

Prevention

As a general precaution it is wise to isolate all new horses as they enter the yard – particularly those from overseas, or the sales ring. Bearing in mind that the incubation period is between one and three days, the horse should remain segregated for this length of time. Similarly, minimize the risk of contact with strange horses; do not allow your animals to come into very close contact with others at shows, meets, etc.

Ideally, all horses should be fully vaccinated; a process that requires both primary and booster vaccinations. This practice is required by all major showgrounds and racecourses, whilst registration of horses with many groups, for example British Eventing, is subject to the horse having a fully completed, up-to-date vaccination certificate. Timing is a factor in the vaccination process. Jockey Club rules (which, in this instance, affect not only racehorses but any horse using racecourse facilities) state that the first two influenza vaccinations should be given not less than 21 days and not more than 92 days apart. In order to comply with this, the first two injections are usually given 4–6 weeks apart. Between 150–215 days after the second injection, a third is given, completing the primary course of vaccination. The rules also state that both primary vaccinations and booster injections must be given at least 10 clear days prior to attending a racecourse.

The first booster is given 6 months after completion of the primary course and from then on normally every 9–12 months. The higher the risk of infection, the more frequently the horse should receive a booster.

Pregnant mares should receive a booster one month before foaling to ensure maximum levels of antibodies. Foals born to fully vaccinated mares will receive antibodies via the colostrum – this protects the foal for the first 3 months of life, after which he will require vaccination. Foals born to unvaccinated mares should be vaccinated earlier than 3 months of age, as should any foal who may be at risk of infection during an epidemic.

Different vaccines provide protection against different strains and provide differing durations of cover. Duvaxyn Plus provides protection against the strains Prague/56, Miami/63 and Suffolk/89. Prevac Pro protects against the strains Prague/56 and Newmarket/93 (American and European-type strain). Equip F provides protection against Newmarket/77, Brentwood/79 and Borlange/91.

Depending upon the type of vaccine used and the vet's advice, the horse should not be subjected to severe exertion following the primary vaccinations; exercise should be light for at least 7 days. This is because the vaccine may give rise to a slight reaction which would be aggravated by strenuous exercise. However, certain vaccines do not carry the requirement for light work after vaccination.

Follow the vet's advice regarding work levels in the days following vaccination. It must be noted that the horse does not gain maximum immunity until 2 weeks after a booster injection.

ITQ 49 List four signs of equine influenza.

1.
2.
3.
4.

ITQ 50 Why is it important that the horse has a long recovery period after suffering from equine influenza?

ITQ 51 What is the procedure for vaccinating foals against equine influenza?

EQUINE HERPES VIRUS

The equine herpes virus can be divided into two subtypes – the **Alpha herpes virus** and the **Beta herpes virus**. The Alpha herpes virus group contains EHV strains 1, 3 and 4, whereas the Beta herpes virus contains EHV 2.

- EHV 1 is the respiratory/abortion strain.
- EHV 2 causes respiratory disease in foals.
- EHV 3 causes venereal disease (coital exanthema virus), an infectious condition resulting in ulcers on the mare's and stallion's genitalia, and occasionally respiratory disease.
- EHV 4 is a respiratory virus (equine rhinopneumonitis).

It is primarily EHV 1 and 4 that affect the respiratory system. Although EHV 1 and 4 are closely related viruses, their DNA structure differs.

The EHV 1 strain can cause abortion in pregnant mares, respiratory problems, or a neurological condition that may lead to paralysis or incoordination. The respiratory condition has an incubation period of between 2–7 days; the abortive condition 2–3 weeks and the neurological condition 7 days.

In the respiratory disease the virus is shed for 2–4 weeks and remains latent throughout the horse's life. Shedding may be activated by stress or corticosteroids.

The horse builds up a level of immunity post-infection, but this is short-lived (2–3 months). Repeated infections may lead to a reduced severity of clinical signs. There is also some cross protection between EHV 1 and 4.

Equine rhinopneumonitis (EHV 4) is a major cause of respiratory disease in horses and is the most common cause of respiratory disease in foals and yearlings. Older horses who show only limited clinical signs may still suffer a loss of performance for up to 3 months. Recovery may be prolonged if the horse continues to work.

Causes

The disease is transmitted through inhalation of the virus released into the air from the respiratory tract of an infected horse or from direct or indirect contact with infective nasal discharge, aborted foetuses or placentas. Infected foals will sometimes carry and spread the virus for up to 9 days while appearing normal; the virus may also remain dormant within an infected horse who appears completely normal (there is no test to detect latent carriers) and may then be activated by stress.

Signs
SIGNS COMMON TO EHV I AND EHV 4

These vary in severity.

- Fever – the temperature will rise to between 102 and 106 °F (39-41 °C), for a period of between 1 and 7 days.
- Watery nasal discharge which becomes purulent if a secondary bacterial infection sets in.
- Disinterest in food and water and general lethargy.
- Occasional coughing – more frequently seen in younger horses after or during exercise – not usually at rest.

- Swollen glands in the throat region.
- If there is a secondary infection clinical signs may persist for 1–2 weeks.

ADDITIONAL SIGNS ASSOCIATED WITH EHV 1

- The neurological strain causes a lack of coordination and possibly paralysis of the hindquarters. Dribbling urine indicates the early stages of incoordination and paralysis.
- Oedema of the throat, neck and lower limbs.
- Infected foals often contract pneumonia. Foals infected neonatally (within the uterus) invariably die.
- An outbreak sometimes causes multiple abortions on a stud.
- When pregnant mares are affected, they may abort approximately three to four weeks after infection (usually in the last trimester). The abortion is sudden, followed by prompt expulsion of the placenta, or the foetus may be delivered in the membranes. The future breeding capacity of the mare is not normally impaired.

ADDITIONAL SIGNS ASSOCIATED WITH EHV 4

- High temperature – up to 41 °C (106 °F).
- Slight clear nasal discharge.
- Enlarged lymph glands.
- Occasional cough.
- May cause the occasional single abortion.

The virus persists in nasal secretions for 20 days. Symptoms may persist for several weeks.

Treatment

1. Call the vet as soon as initial signs are noticed. Nasopharyngeal swabs will be taken to give a positive identification of the virus. Any aborted foetus and placenta should be sent for post-mortem examination.

2. Adhere to strict rules of isolation. Steam-clean and disinfect any affected stable and burn all bedding.

3. Ensure that the horse has plenty of fresh air and complete rest.

4. The vet will prescribe antibiotics, **mucolytics** (drugs which aid the breakdown and clearance of mucus) and bronchodilators as necessary.

5. Prevent all movement of horses in and out of the yard. Keep all other stock away from pregnant mares.

The Horserace Betting Levy Board has prepared a Code of Practice for the United Kingdom and Ireland with regard to all aspects of EHV 1. If EHV 1 is confirmed, the appropriate breeders' association should be informed.

Immunity

The horse will acquire a certain degree of immunity following infection. A live vaccine may be administered although, where breeding stock are concerned, it is usual to use a killed vaccine for fear of reversion to virulence. Pregnant mares may be administered killed viral vaccine (**Pneumabort K**) in months five, seven and nine of pregnancy to help prevent abortions. All horses on the premises should be vaccinated as a preventative measure. Two doses of vaccine are given 3–4 weeks apart, followed by a booster 6 months later, then annually.

ITQ 52 There are four strains of equine herpes virus.

a. Which type most commonly causes mares to abort?

b. What clinical signs occur with both EHV 1 and EHV 4?

c. How is EHV 1 transmitted?

ITQ 53 What is the procedure for vaccinating pregnant mares against EHV 1?

EQUINE VIRAL ARTERITIS (EVA)

Also referred to as 'pink eye', this disease was introduced to the United Kingdom by a Polish stallion in 1993. It causes acute respiratory infection and is significant amongst breeding stock as it also causes abortion.

Such is the impact of EVA, it is a notifiable disease. This means that, under the Animal Health Act 1981 the Divisional Veterinary Manager (DVM) of the Department for Environment, Food and Rural Affairs (Defra) must be notified as soon as the disease is suspected.

Causes

The virus can be transmitted as a result of venereal infection of mares by stallions during covering, via semen during artificial insemination (AI), via droplet infection (coughing and snorting) and through direct contact with saliva, nasal secretions, blood, aborted foetuses and the products of an abortion or parturition.

Signs

The signs vary in severity and may include one or more of the following:
- Loss of appetite and depression.

- Watery nasal discharge, which may later become purulent.
- Fever – temperature rise to 106 °F which may persist for up to 12 days.
- Sometimes coughing and respiratory distress.
- Mucous membranes become reddened and the eyes become inflamed (hence the name 'pink eye').
- Oedema of hind limbs, scrotum or udder.
- Abortion occurs simultaneously with symptoms, thus distinguishing it from rhinopneumonitis.
- Leucopenia (reduced white blood cells in circulation).

Some infected horses show no signs.

Treatment

There is no treatment for the disease itself but the following should happen if EVA occurs:

1. Seek veterinary advice and notify the Divisional Veterinary Manager of Defra.
2. Stop movement on and off the premises.
3. Stop mating and teasing.
4. Stop semen collection for AI.
5. Isolate clinical cases and horses known to have been in contact.
6. All horses on the premises must be screened by blood testing and segregated accordingly.
7. Blood tests should be repeated at 14-day intervals until the outbreak is over.

Full information is given in the Horserace Betting Levy Board's Code of Practice.

Prevention

1. Vaccinate using **Artervac**. Vaccinated horses become seropositive, so their EVA seronegative status must be determined before vaccination.
2. Breeding stock must be confirmed free of EVA before mating, collection of semen for AI and prior to arrival at stud to foal.
3. Stallions can be permanent carriers and shed the virus in their semen. Tests will be carried out on seropositive stallions whilst under strict isolation. This involves testing the semen for virus; if the test is negative, it is followed by two test matings. If the mares remain seronegative following mating the stallion is unlikely to be a shedder. Shedder stallions must be castrated (followed by 6 weeks isolation), or euthanased.

BACTERIAL INFECTIONS OF THE RESPIRATORY TRACT
STRANGLES

This highly infectious and contagious condition affects the upper respiratory tract. Young animals are very susceptible to strangles, but it affects horses of all ages. In a susceptible population morbidity will reach 100 per cent, however mortality is low (1–5 per cent).

Causes

Strangles is caused by the bacterium *Streptococcus equi*. Bacteria are expelled into the air when an infected horse coughs; the nasal discharges and discharge from an abscess are also extremely infective. The obvious sources of infection are thus either direct contact with a diseased animal or inhalation of infective air, but contact with infected woodwork is another cause that must be taken seriously. This is because the bacteria present in pus from a strangles abscess may remain infective within structures such as stables and wooden fencing for many months.

Signs

The incubation period (period between becoming infected and showing the first signs) is generally between 3 and 8 days, although it may extend up to 14 days. The first sign is disinterest in taking food or water. This is followed by:

- Fever – a rise in temperature, which may go as high as 41.5 °C (105 °F).
- Watery nasal discharge, which becomes thick and pus-like. This may be from one or both nostrils.
- A soft, moist cough.
- Slight increase in respiratory rate.
- The horse may stand with his neck distended.
- The lymph glands in the throat region become swollen and the horse may experience difficulty in swallowing.
- Abscesses may form at the site of the lymph glands. These become hot, tense and painful and will eventually mature, burst and drain.

The vet will confirm the diagnosis by taking swabs from the nasal discharge or exudate from the abscesses.

Other Forms of Strangles

In a more chronic form, the condition is known as **bastard strangles**. This is not epidemic in nature, affecting only individual horses. The signs include fever, and abscesses that may appear in different areas of the body. Superficial swellings burst without complication but if the swellings interfere with breathing, this form of the disease can lead to death.

An atypical form of strangles has recently been observed where there exists a transient fever, modest nasal discharge and slightly raised lymph nodes. It is thought that this particular strain may have arisen because of infection of partially immune animals or as a result of a less virulent strain.

Treatment and Control

Keep the horse warm and adhere to strict isolation rules. If the infected horse has been turned out there is a risk that the paddock has been infected. It should be rested and all other horses who have been grazing it should be isolated. The field will be infective for at least 4 weeks.

The rectal temperature of the sick horse should be monitored. If the temperature rises, antibiotics should be administered. Antibiotics, in particular penicillin, are effective against *Streptocccus equi*. Early, prompt and continued treatment may prevent abscess formation. However, in the later stages of this condition, antibiotic therapy may delay the maturing and bursting of the abscesses. In such instances, antibiotics are often withheld until the abscesses have ruptured.

Hot fomentation of abscesses will help them to mature; once mature they may be surgically drained. At this point the healing process is more noticeable as the horse starts to show signs of recovery. Remove purulent discharges with non-irritating antiseptic solution and flush out the ruptured or lanced abscesses twice daily with a dilute solution of hydrogen peroxide or Pevidene.

Twice daily inhalations of eucalyptus oil or Friar's Balsam can ease congestion of the upper respiratory tract.

The vet may also administer a non-steroidal anti-inflammatory drug, e.g. phenylbutazone, to lower the temperature and reduce the pain and swelling, which often leads to an improved appetite. While the horse is unwell, feed only soft mashes.

In cases where the horse is having severe difficulties breathing, (dyspnoea), a temporary tracheotomy may be required.

As this condition is often severely debilitating, the horse will need a very long period of rest. Infected horses should be kept in isolation for at least 6–8 weeks after the last of the symptoms disappear.

Prevention

Prevention focuses on isolation procedures. In addition, new horses entering yards should be quarantined for 2 weeks before mixing with other horses.

There is also a strangles vaccine that can be administered through a submucosal injection in the upper lip. The level of risk influences the frequency of vaccination: following an initial vaccination of two injections, 4 weeks apart, high-risk horses need to be vaccinated thereafter every 3 months, medium-risk horses every 6 months.

ITQ 54

a. Name the microbe that causes strangles.

b. Give three signs of strangles.
1.
2.
3.

ITQ 55 When a horse is suffering from strangles, at what point is the vet likely to administer antibiotics?

LARYNGITIS AND TRACHEITIS

These bacterial infections of the upper respiratory tract cause inflammation of the larynx or trachea. They may occur singly or together.

Signs

- Difficulty in swallowing.
- Laboured breathing.
- Coughing.
- Rise in temperature.

Treatment

1. Call the vet, who may administer antibiotics.
2. Dampen all feed well – give mashes and gruels.
3. Keep the horse warm but ensure plenty of fresh air and follow general rules of sick nursing.

SINUSITIS

This is a bacterial infection within one of the sinuses, causing inflammation of the membranous lining and the accumulation of pus.

Although the sinuses are not directly involved in the process of respiration, their infection may be secondary to a viral or bacterial respiratory disorder and signs are closely associated to those of the upper respiratory tract. In some cases, however, the secondary infection may arise from a damaged tooth root.

Signs

- Greyish nasal discharge, normally from one nostril.
- Swollen, tender area around sinus – normally just beneath the eye. Percussion (gentle tapping with a finger), in this area will show a reaction.

Treatment

1. The vet may drain the sinus surgically and administer antibiotics.
2. The sinus will need to be flushed daily.
3. If present, an infected tooth root will be treated. If the tooth is abnormal it will be removed.

RESPIRATORY CONDITIONS OF VIRAL, BACTERIAL, OR OTHER ORIGIN

PNEUMONIA

This serious condition causes inflammation of the lung tissue and, in cases of bronchopneumonia, the bronchi. Foals, especially those under 6 months old, are particularly susceptible to bacterial pneumonia and may become very ill.

Causes

- Bacterial, viral or fungal infection.
- Pneumonia may also occur as a secondary infection to equine influenza or,

particularly in foals, inherited immuno-deficiency.

- In foals under 6 months of age *Rhodococcus equi* causes **summer pneumonia**.
- Newborn foals may become infected through the navel – the bacteria circulate through the body and reach the lungs.
- Parasitic damage.

Signs

- Coughing.
- An increase in temperature – 39.5–41 °C (103–106 °F).
- Increased rate of pulse and respiration.
- Respiratory distress: laboured breathing, abnormal sound – a moist rattle and bronchial sounds, flared nostrils and a double expiratory effort (heaves).
- There may be mucopurulent discharge in the trachea and at the nostrils.
- The horse will appear very cold and tucked up, with a poor appetite.
- In the case of foal pneumonia the abdominal lymph nodes may develop abscesses.

Treatment

1. Isolate and immediately seek and follow veterinary advice. The vet may administer a combination of antibiotics, bronchodilators and mucolytics.
2. Very sick horses will require pain relief, fluid therapy and possibly oxygen.
3. Keep the horse warm – with rugs and possibly heat lamps – and provide plenty of draught-free fresh air.

ITQ 56

a. What causes pneumonia?

b. Which microbe frequently causes summer pneumonia in foals?

BRONCHITIS

This is an inflammatory condition which normally affects the bronchi but can also affect the bronchioles – in which case it is known as **bronchiolitis**.

Causes

Very often these conditions are secondary to another infection. If the infection is bacterial or viral, the disease may be transmitted. Any infection and/or reactions to dust, allergens such as smoke or irritant gases, etc. can cause bronchitis as part of the disease process; it is part of many disease conditions affecting the respiratory tract.

Signs

- Coughing spasms – the cough may persist for 2–3 weeks.

- Bilateral nasal discharge.
- A slight rise in temperature.
- A generally dull, depressed state.
- When the bronchitis is caused through bacterial infection, examination by endoscope may show mucopurulent exudate in the trachea.

Treatment

1. The vet may administer antibiotics to treat bacterial infection, and also mucolytic drugs.

2. Adhere to the general rules of sick nursing; complete rest, plenty of fresh air, a dust-free environment. Keep the horse warm and feed soft, easily swallowed and digestible food.

GENERAL VIRAL DISEASES
EQUINE INFECTIOUS ANAEMIA

This highly infectious disease, also known as swamp fever, is endemic (occurs in small groups of animals) in the western states of America, the north-western states of Canada, Europe, Asia and Africa. The first case in Britain was reported in 1975 and more recently there have been outbreaks in Northern Ireland and the Republic of Ireland. Equine infectious anaemia (EIA) is a notifiable disease – if a horse is suspected of being affected a Divisional Veterinary Manager of Defra must be notified.

Causes

EIA is caused by a very resistant virus which is capable of remaining in the blood for many years. The virus is transmitted via biting insects such as horseflies and mosquitoes, contaminated syringes and needles, or through contact with infective urine, faeces, saliva, nasal discharge, semen or milk.

Signs
ACUTE FORM

- Fever – temperature rises to between 40–42 ºC (105 ºF).
- Anaemia.
- Weight loss.
- Depression.
- Weakness.
- Infection of pregnant mares may lead to abortion, stillbirth or birth of a weak foal.

SUBACUTE FORM

- Fever for 1–7 days. The temperature intermittently returns to normal.
- Loss of appetite.
- Weight loss.
- Depression.
- Jaundice.

CHRONIC FORM

- Initial weight loss after which the horse regains some condition and appears 'normal'. However, the virus is still present in the blood.

Treatment

There is no specific treatment other than supportive therapy on humane grounds prior to euthanasia.

Control

1. There is no vaccine to prevent EIA.
2. Affected horses must be euthanased.
3. Horses should not be moved from endemic areas. Any who are imported from countries known to have the disease must be blood-sampled for testing. This test is referred to as the Coggin's test.
4. The number of insect carriers should be reduced with insecticides and repellents.
5. All needles and syringes must be clean.
6. Any horse suspected of infection must be isolated for at least 45 days, but preferably 90 days.

ITQ 57

a. In which countries is equine infectious anaemia endemic?

b. How is this disease transmitted?

EQUINE ENCEPHALOMYELITIS

There are several strains of this notifiable disease, seen mainly in North and South America, Russia and the Far and Middle East.

Causes

The viruses are insect-borne, varying in virulence but all producing the same clinical signs.

Signs

- Fever.
- Loss of appetite and condition.
- Depression.
- Drowsiness followed by violent excitability.
- Paralysis.
- Incoordination.
- Collapse followed by death.

Diagnosis may prove difficult – laboratory confirmation is necessary to identify the strain of virus. The signs may be confused with rabies, botulism, leptospirosis or African horse sickness.

Treatment

Although the mortality rate varies between strains, this disease is very often fatal. The most dangerous strain, with a 90 per cent mortality rate, may be passed on to humans. There is very little that can be done by way of effective treatment, but a vaccination exists (see Control).

Control

1. Annual vaccination. Pregnant mares need to be given a booster 4–6 weeks before foaling.
2. Stable the horse at night.
3. Use repellents to deter insects.

GENERAL BACTERIAL DISEASES
MUD FEVER
Causes

If horses are left standing in a wet and muddy field for long periods, the bacteria *Dermatophilus congolensis* in the mud enter the pores of the skin, causing an infection.

Brushing wet mud into the skin aggravates the condition.

Signs

- The skin on the back of the horse's legs (and sometimes the stomach) becomes inflamed. The condition is also referred to as **dermatitis** for this reason.
- The skin will crack and serum will exude.
- The horse will be in pain and in severe cases he will be lame.
- The lower limbs may be swollen.

Treatment

1. Remove the horse from the muddy field.
2. Using curved scissors, clip away the hair from the affected area.
3. Wash the legs thoroughly with a mild antibacterial wash such as Hibiscrub to remove scabs and debris, rinse thoroughly and pat dry carefully with a clean towel.
4. Apply an anti-bacterial, anti-inflammatory preparation and keep the horse stabled.
5. Apply stable bandages over clean Gamgee to keep the area clean and prevent bedding from sticking to the treated area.
6. If the skin is badly infected the vet must be called to administer antibiotics and the area may need to be poulticed using Animalintex. The Animalintex can be warm and wet at first – this will draw out infection and prevent excessive drying of the skin, which would exacerbate the problem of cracking. Once the infection has been bought under control the dressing can be left off and the area treated with an anti-bacterial cream.

7. Check that the horse is up to date with his tetanus vaccinations as the tetanus bacteria are found in the soil and could enter through the broken skin.

8. If the condition does not improve with better management, consult the vet.

Prevention

- Avoid turning horses out in wet, muddy fields if possible.
- If the horse has to stay out in a muddy field, rub liquid paraffin or Vaseline into the skin on his legs to help waterproof the skin.
- Try to improve the muddy areas, for example around the gate, in your paddock.
- Never brush wet mud as this pushes the mud particles into the skin.

TETANUS (LOCKJAW)
Cause

Clostridium tetani is picked up from the soil via an open wound. *Clostridium tetani* is an anaerobe, which means it thrives only in the absence of oxygen. Once within a wound, especially a deep puncture wound, the bacteria proliferate and produce a very potent toxin that is then absorbed into the circulatory system. From thereon it affects the central nervous system, causing distressing symptoms.

Signs

- Loss of appetite and desire to drink.
- Gradually worsening stiffness, muscle tremors and reluctance to move.
- The forelegs may be splayed and the head and neck outstretched, possibly with the head and tail raised.
- Raising the head and tapping the chin causes the third eyelid to pass over the eye.
- Sudden sound or exposure to light may send the horse into violent spasms.
- The jaws become clamped.
- No urine or faeces will be passed.
- The horse may become recumbent and be unable to rise.
- Death occurs if the respiratory muscles are affected.

Treatment

1. Consult the vet immediately.
2. Adhere to the rules of sick nursing, keep the horse in a quiet, darkened stable and follow the vet's advice.
3. This condition is usually fatal, although large doses of antibiotics and tetanus antitoxin may be effective if administered early enough.

Prevention

Tetanus toxoid is used to immunize horses against tetanus. It is a 'detoxified' toxin and causes an immune response to be built up for protection against the toxin itself. Tetanus vaccination is extremely effective. The recommended regime is two doses 4–6 weeks apart (usually in conjunction with the 'flu vaccination), then after one year, then every two years. Vaccination more frequently than once a year is not generally recommended.

Foals may be vaccinated at 3 months of age. Before this, protection may be given using the antitoxin, as the immune system is not mature enough to respond to vaccination. Tetanus antitoxin binds to any circulating toxin and neutralizes it. It will protect an unvaccinated animal for approximately three to four weeks, and is used when a horse of uncertain vaccinal status sustains an injury or is at risk from tetanus infection, for example when foaling. It does not, however give long-term protection. The toxoid can be given at the same time, provided different injection sites are used.

Pregnant mares should be vaccinated with tetanus toxoid one month before the anticipated foaling date to ensure that high levels of protective antibodies are passed to the foal via the colostrum.

LEPTOSPIROSIS

This infectious disease affects both horses and humans, although it is more common in dogs than either horses or humans. In the horse, leptospirosis is usually a mild disease with a good prognosis. In humans, it can be fatal.

Cause

It is caused by the bacteria *Leptospira interrogans serovers*. These microbes are generally water-borne and infection may occur as a result of contact with infective urine or urine-contaminated feed. The most common cause is rodents infecting feedstuffs. (In humans, the inhalation of urinary vapours can lead to infection.) Fairly recently (1999) flooding in the USA has caused leptospirosis which resulted in equine abortion. Following infection, the bacteria (leptospires) often accumulate in the kidneys and are shed in the urine for a long time.

Signs
- Rise in temperature: 39.5–40.5 °C (103–105 °F).
- Depression and dullness.
- Loss of appetite and condition.
- Jaundice symptoms.
- Possible abortion in pregnant mares.
- Inflammation of the iris, ciliary body and choroid of the eyeball. (This condition is known as **periodic ophthalmia** or **moon blindness**, and is an intermittent recurrent disease that can eventually lead to blindness.)

Treatment

The vet will administer antibiotics – penicillin and streptomycin are effective. The prognosis is generally good, although the disease can be fatal in foals.

ITQ 58

a. Which microbe causes leptospirosis?

b. Name and describe the eye condition that may accompany leptospirosis.

BOTULISM
Causes
This condition is caused by the toxins of the bacteria *Clostridium botulinum*, which are present in the soil and are a fairly common contaminant of animal feedstuffs. However, although contamination of feedstuff by rats is one cause of botulism, the condition had not been reported frequently in horses until big bale silage and haylage started to be used as equine forage.

To understand the most likely cause of botulism in horses, it is necessary to know something of the process by which grass crops are converted into silage and haylage.

Since all bovines can cope with *Clostridium botulinum*, farmers have traditionally cut low for silage, but grass crops cut too low will contain the bacteria. Once the crop is bagged, if the fermentation process is interrupted or compromised, these may proliferate and produce the toxins that cause botulism. This is more likely to happen with silage than with haylage, both because silage is cut 'greener' (earlier) and lower than haylage and because responsible producers of the latter are aware of the need to supply a product suitable for horses.

Signs
- General weakness.
- Difficulty in eating.
- Progressive paralysis which results in the horse moving with a shuffling, stiff gait, dragging his toes along the ground.
- Horse may stand with his head and neck distended.
- Respiratory paralysis may occur, resulting in death.
- Where big bale silage is implicated, because of the size of the bales, a number of horses may be affected.

Treatment
1. The vet will administer an antitoxin; even so, the prognosis is guarded.
2. Fluids and electrolytes may be administered via a stomach tube – this has proved helpful in the small number of cases that have survived.

Prevention
- Horses must be introduced very gradually to silage and great care must be taken that it is not contaminated. If in any doubt, silage is best avoided as forage for horses.

- Haylage should never be used if the sealing of the bag has been damaged and, once a bag has been opened, the contents should be used quickly, within the terms on the manufacturer's label.

SALMONELLOSIS
Causes

There are over a thousand different types of bacteria in the salmonella group, of which approximately forty may affect horses. Of these, it is most frequently *Salmonella typhimurium* which causes the disease in the horse. Anything contaminated with faecal matter will cause the disease to spread, e.g. pasture, feedstuffs, and drinking water.

This bacterium is infectious to humans, so great attention must be paid to hygiene when nursing sick horses.

Signs

Salmonellosis generally occurs in four forms.

PERACUTE

This form mainly affects foals. The signs, which arise suddenly, are:
- Temperature rise to 40–41 °C (104–106 °F).
- Depression and weakness.
- Loss of appetite.
- Increased heart rate and weak pulse.
- Increased respiratory rate.
- Blueing of mucous membranes.
- Abdominal pain and diarrhoea, with the latter leading to dehydration and electrolyte imbalance.
- Death usually occurs within 72 hours.

ACUTE

This form mainly affects adult horses. The signs appear suddenly and include:
- Temperature rise to 40–41 °C (104–106 °F).
- Depression and weakness.
- Loss of appetite.
- Increased heart rate and weakened pulse.
- Increased respiratory rate.
- Diarrhoea – this sometimes does not develop for a few days but then leads to dehydration and electrolyte imbalance.

Some horses survive, and of those that do, some:
— Recover fully and are not carriers.
— Become asymptomatic carriers but never shed the organisms.
— Become asymptomatic carriers and shed intermittently or continually.
— Become chronic cases.

CHRONIC

Signs that may continue in survivors of the acute form include:

- Often, damage to the intestinal lining.
- Loss of condition.
- Possible loss of appetite.
- Soft faeces and diarrhoea.

The horse may still die eventually, or have to be destroyed.

ATYPICAL

This may occur after a stressful situation such as transportation, competition or undergoing surgery. Signs include:

- High temperature: 39.5–41 °C (103–106 °F).
- Loss of appetite.
- Depression.
- Mild abdominal pain.
- Soft faeces.

The horse generally recovers within a few days.

Treatment

1. The vet will confirm the diagnosis of salmonellosis through the results of faecal culture.
2. Anti-endotoxic drugs, e.g. flunixin will be administered.
3. Fluid and electrolyte therapy is essential to combat dehydration.
4. Plasma, blood or plasma volume expander therapy may be needed.
5. Antibiotics may be prescribed in certain cases. (As toxins are more of a problem, antibiotics are not often prescribed).
6. The horse must be kept in isolation.

Those handling the sick horse must wear overalls and rubber gloves while handling the horse and pay great attention to hygiene afterwards, e.g. arm and hand scrubbing, boot dipping. The overalls, gloves and boots should be worn when handling the sick horse only.

> ITQ 59
>
> a. Which microbe most commonly causes salmonellosis in the horse?
>
> b. What is 'atypical salmonellosis' and how is it caused?

CONTAGIOUS EQUINE METRITIS (CEM)

This highly contagious bacterial venereal disease is a serious threat to breeding stock as it causes greatly reduced rates of conception. It was first diagnosed and identified in Great Britain in 1977, before which it was unheard of.

Because of its effect on fertility, CEM is a notifiable disease. If suspected, a report must be made to the Local Divisional Veterinary Manager of Defra and, upon confirmation of a diagnosis in Great Britain, The Thoroughbred Breeders' Association at Newmarket must be notified.

Causes

The CEM microbe, *Taylorella equigenitalis*, is found mainly around the area of the clitoris, cervix and urethra in the mare. Stallions may carry the organisms over the surface of the penis and in the urethral fossa, but show no clinical signs of the disease.

Infection can occur:

1. During nose to genital contact prior to covering or during teasing.
2. During covering via genital to genital contact. If the mare is infected around the clitoral and cervical area, covering or manual examination may push the organisms forward into the uterus, causing endometritis* (inflammation of the lining of the uterus).
3. Through contaminated water, utensils and instruments.
4. On the hands of staff and veterinary surgeons who handle the tail and genital area of the mare or the penis of the stallion.

Signs

In some mares, there may be no obvious signs: others show a profuse purulent discharge from the vulva. This usually occurs 1–6 days after infection.

Treatment

1. If CEM is confirmed in mares prior to mating, infected mares must be isolated and treated as advised by the vet. All owners who have booked mares to any stallion, or whose mares have recently left the stud, must be notified.
2. Penicillin may be administered by intrauterine infusion and/or intramuscular injection.
3. If CEM is confirmed after mating the above procedure must again be followed. In addition, the stallion should cease covering mares and must be swabbed and treated as advised by the vet. Covering should not resume until the stallion has been treated and has had three negative sets of swabs.
4. The first swab should not be taken until at least 7 days after the completion of treatment and subsequent swabs should be taken at intervals of not less than 2 days. The stallion should then be test-mated to at least three mares, who are swabbed afterwards. All mares implicated must be checked – this may include blood tests.

---

*Endometritis leads to infertility as it causes the early resorption of the hormone-producing corpus luteum. This results in the mare repeatedly coming back into season at shorter intervals than normal, or 'short-cycling'.

Prevention
SWABBING PROCEDURES

Swabbing is a quick and efficient method of assessing the presence of bacterial contamination within the reproductive tract of both mare and stallion. It is an essential practice for the following reasons:

- Mucosal secretions may be tested for the presence of pathogenic organisms.

- It prevents the transmission of venereal bacteria from the stallion's genitalia to that of the mare, or vice versa.

- It assists in the detection of endometritis, thus helping to optimize fertility.

Swabs are therefore taken as part of the preventative routine at all studs in accordance with the 'Common Codes of Practice for the Control of Contagious Equine Metritis and other Equine Bacterial Venereal Diseases and Equine Viral Arteritis'. The Codes are published by the Horserace Betting Levy Board and apply to the breeding season in Canada, France, Germany, Italy, Ireland, the USA and the UK. The Codes are reviewed and re-published annually and are available from the Thoroughbred Breeders' Association, Stanstead House, The Avenue, Newmarket, Suffolk, UK or from the Defra website at www.defra.gov.uk.

Regarding contagious equine metritis, mares are defined in the Codes of Practice as being either 'high risk' or 'low risk'. The following are defined as 'high risk':

- All mares from whom the contagious equine metritis organism (CEMO) has been isolated in the last two years.

- Any mare covered/teased by a stallion/teaser who transmitted CEM the previous year.

- All mares arriving from countries other than Canada, France, Germany, Ireland, Italy, the USA and the UK, if covered by stallions resident outside these countries in the previous year.

- Barren and maiden mares arriving from countries other than Canada, France, Germany, Ireland, Italy, the USA or the UK.

All mares not defined as 'high risk' are designated 'low risk', and are subject to less stringent testing than the 'high risk' mares. Should a mare be covered in Canada, France, Germany, Ireland, Italy, the USA or the UK, then return to another country and subsequently come back to one of the participating countries, she will be regarded as 'low risk' provided she has not been covered in a 'high risk' country in the interim.

	TYPE OF SWAB	WHEN	WHERE
'Low risk' mares	Clitoral	Prior to arrival at stud or on arrival	Home (by agreement with stud manager) Stud
	Endometrial	During oestrus prior to covering Repeated in subsequent oestrus if not in foal	Stud
'High risk' mares	Clitoral	First: before arrival at stud Second: after arrival Third: during oestrus	Home Stud Stud
	Endometrial	During oestrus Repeated in subsequent oestrus if not in foal	Stud

Table 1 Summary of swabbing procedure

CERTIFICATION

This confirms that mares and stallions have been tested free of CEM.

The mare's certificate is completed by the mare's owner and lodged with the prospective stallion's owner or stud manager before the mare is sent to the stud. The certificate should include the following information.

- Name of mare.
- Passport number.
- Owner's name and address.
- Details of studs visited, previous coverings and outcomes.

Additional information, including results of positive bacteriological examinations for CEMO, *Klebsiella pneumoniae* (including capsule type – see Laboratory Certificate, opposite) and *Pseudomonas aeruginosa.*

The stallion's certificate is a certificate of examination of the stallion, to be completed by a veterinary surgeon. It should contain the following information:

- Name of stallion.
- Passport number.
- The two dates upon which swabs were obtained from the penile sheath, urethra, urethral fossa and a sample of pre-ejaculatory fluid.
- Name of the Designated Laboratory.
- Confirmation of negative results.
- Name, address and signature of the veterinary surgeon responsible.

The laboratory certificate is issued only by a 'Designated Laboratory' – one whose name is published in the *Veterinary Record* by the Horserace Betting Levy Board. The certificate should include the following information:

- Name of stallion or mare the swabs were taken from (as labelled on transport medium container).
- Sites swabs taken from.
- Who submitted swabs.
- Date that swabs were bacteriologically examined.
- Name and qualifications of person responsible for examination.
- Name of laboratory.
- Confirmation that CEMO, *Klebsiella pneumoniae* or *Pseudomonas aeruginosa* was or was not isolated. (If *pneumoniae* was isolated, the capsule type must be stated. Only types KI, 2 and 5 are venereal pathogens.)

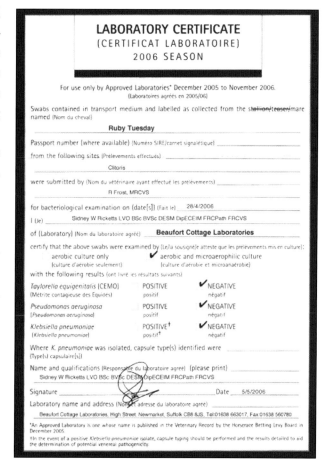

Figure 16 The laboratory certificate

Covering should not take place until the relevant certificates, confirming negative results, are received.

ITQ 60

a. Which microbe causes contagious equine metritis?

b. How is CEM transmitted?

c. Why is CEM a serious threat to breeding stock?

INFECTIOUS SKIN CONDITIONS
RINGWORM
Causes

Ringworm is a fungal infection of the skin caused by dermaphytic (skin 'loving') fungi *Trichophyton spp.* and *Microsporum spp.* As it is contagious it is passed on by indirect contact with infected grooming kit, tack and clothing as well as by direct contact. *It can also be passed on to humans.*

Some cattle may have ringworm and the fungus can remain potentially active within structures, e.g. woodwork, for many years.

Signs

- Round and/or irregular patches of raised hair (tufts) appear anywhere on the body but most frequently on the head, neck, girth and saddle areas.
- Beneath the tufts, the skin may ooze fluid (exudate), although sometimes the lesions are dry and scaly from the start.
- The tufts stick together in a crust of exudate before falling out.
- After approximately four weeks the hair will regrow.
- The incubation period is 7–14 days.

Treatment and Prevention of Spread

Wear rubber or disposable gloves when handling infected horses. Wash hands thoroughly after treatment. Overalls should be worn to protect clothing.

1. Isolate the horse and keep grooming kit, rugs, numnahs, etc. separate.
2. Wash all grooming kit in a fungicidal solution.
3. Stop grooming the affected horse as this spreads the infection.
4. Use a summer sheet beneath stable and turnout rugs as this can be easily washed. Soak the sheet in fungicide approximately twice a week.
5. Apply iodine lotion (Pevidine) to patches and carefully dispose of the cotton wool afterwards. Never apply near the eyes as iodine will cause severe irritation.
6. The vet may prescribe griseofulvin – an anti-fungal powder which is mixed in with the feed.
7. Burn bedding and steam-clean and disinfect stables with a suitable fungicide. Creosote all wooden structures
8. Do not transport infected horses as the lorry or trailer will become contaminated.

After recovery, horses develop an immunity that lasts for several months.

RAIN SCALD
Causes

Excessive soaking of the skin through prolonged exposure to driving rain causes the skin to becomes softened, allowing the bacteria *Dermotophilus congolensis* to penetrate. This leads to dermatitis.

Signs

- Tufts of hair become matted together. The tufts can be lifted off along with a thick crust of exudate.
- Beneath the tufts the skin may be dry or it may exude serum.
- Rain scald most commonly affects the shoulders, back, loins and quarters.

Since these signs are broadly similar to ringworm, it may be necessary to consult the vet for confirmation of the condition.

Treatment

1. Stable the horse if possible.
2. Gently remove the tufts either by hand or by using a fine-toothed metal comb.
3. If exudate is present, clean the area with Hibiscrub.
4. In severe cases consult the vet, as antibiotics may be needed.
5. Once healed, use a turnout rug to prevent the skin from getting soaked again.

CHAPTER SUMMARY

This chapter has dealt with the main infectious diseases of the horse. It is not, however, an exhaustive study of equine infectious disease, and the depth at which the diseases have been described gives only a layperson's (as opposed to a veterinary surgeon's) level of knowledge. Therefore, the vet must be consulted is a horse is unwell.

So far we have looked mainly at infectious diseases – we'll look next at some of the non-infectious diseases.

CHAPTER 5

NON-INFECTIOUS DISEASES

The aims and objectives of this chapter are to explain:

- The signs, causes and treatments of metabolic disorders.
- The signs, causes and treatment of disorders of the gastrointestinal tract.

METABOLIC DISORDERS
EQUINE EXERTIONAL RHABDOMYOLYSIS (EER)

This is the name now used by the veterinary profession to describe any condition that involves muscle breakdown. Other terms that are, or have been, used to describe this condition, or particular aspects of it, include:

- Azoturia.
- Tying-up syndrome.
- Setfast.
- Monday morning disease.
- Paralytic/equine myoglobinuria.
- Blackwater.
- Exertional myopathy.

Causes

The exact cause of EER is not fully understood and it is subject to ongoing research. However, it is generally considered that the following can trigger an attack:

- A deficiency in, or imbalance of, vitamin E, selenium, salts and electrolytes can affect the normal function of nerves and muscles. This may occur as a result of significant sweat losses in sports such as eventing or endurance riding.

- Enforced box rest on normal working rations, particularly if these rations are high in carbohydrates.

- Irregular exercise of a fit horse.

- Sudden stressful situations, e.g. crashing in to a showjump. In wild ungulates the sudden stress of being caught and confined leads to a similar condition termed **capture myopathy**.

- Since there is a high incidence in mares it is thought there may possibly be a hormonal link.

- There are examples of offspring inheriting the tendency to 'tie up'.

- Defects/abnormalities in polysaccharide (glycogen) storage in muscle cells.

Signs

This condition most usually affects the fit, stabled horse upon return to work after a period of enforced rest.

- The horse works normally at first but, a short while later, is reluctant to move. In mild cases the muscles of the hindquarters become stiff and tense but improve with gentle walking. This is frequently known as 'tying-up'.

- The horse may stagger, sweat profusely and show signs of quickened breathing. This indicates that the condition is more serious.

- In very severe cases the hindquarters are so painful and tense that the horse cannot stand. If the horse is made to move, the hocks and fetlocks become flexed and the hindquarters sink.

- Repeated attempts to urinate. Any urine passed will be a much darker colour than normal (reddish-brown to almost black) and will have a strange smell. This is caused by release of the pigment myoglobin when muscle fibres are destroyed. Myoglobin is then excreted in the urine.

- Increased heart rate and respiration.

- Mild colicky signs when the horse stands still.

Treatment

1. Immediate action whilst out on exercise is to dismount, slacken the girth and cover the hindquarters with a jacket or rug. Then call for assistance and box home.

2. Do not force the horse to walk as this can lead to increased muscle damage.

3. If the condition is very severe call the vet, who will advise on transporting the horse home. Some surgeries have a horse ambulance or specially converted trailer. A horse who cannot stand is obviously in need of specialist equipment to facilitate transportation.

4. Keep the horse warm while waiting for transport to be organized.

5. Once home, if you have not already done so, call the vet. Place warm blankets over the quarters to help relax the muscles. If they are installed, infrared lamps provide warmth. (These must be securely installed with all wires safely encased.) Ensure that the horse cannot touch the lamps and that no bedding or clothing can come into contact with them.

6. Diet should be changed to include only hay, water and, if necessary, low-energy horse and pony cubes. High-energy cubes (with high carbohydrate levels) must be avoided.

7. The vet may give an anti-inflammatory analgesic such as phenylbutazone.

8. The dark colour in the urine is, as mentioned, myoglobin released from the damaged muscle cells. Myoglobin is a large molecule that impairs the filtration system and thus can damage the kidneys. In severe cases, fluids may have to be administered to flush the pigment from the kidneys.

9. Blood testing for levels of muscle enzymes CK (creatine kinase) and AST (aspartate aminotransferase) will help to determine the severity of an attack.

10. Rest is essential – the length of the rest period will depend upon the severity of the attack, but at all times the vet's advice should be followed. If the horse is worked too soon, further muscle damage may occur.

Prevention

Once a horse has suffered from EER he will always be prone to further attacks. Preventative action is of great importance.

1. Feed according to the work done. Some of the energy may be provided in the form of fats rather than carbohydrates.

2. Always feed a well-balanced diet. Reduce carbohydrates whenever possible and ensure a balance of electrolytes, vitamin E and selenium.

3. Keep feed ahead of work – cut back onto a low carbohydrate diet the day before a rest day.

4. Follow a careful fitness programme so that the horse's muscles are never overstressed, and follow a regular pattern of exercise.

5. On rest days a horse prone to this condition should not stand in his stable; either lead out in hand or turn out for a few hours.

ITQ 61 Give two of the names by which equine exertional rhabdomyolysis (EER) is also known.

1.

2.

ITQ 62 Why is the urine a dark reddish-brown after an attack of EER?

ITQ 63 State two possible causes of EER.

1.

2.

ITQ 64 List three signs of EER.

1.
2.
3.

ITQ 65 What immediate action should be taken if a horse is suspected of having 'tied up'?

HYPERLIPAEMIA
Causes

This condition is caused by abnormally high levels of lipids in the blood and can be seen in starved horses who are not receiving sufficient food to meet their energy requirements. The reduced food intake leads to a breakdown of adipose tissue to compensate. The liver uses some of this fat to produce energy but, if the energy deficiency is prolonged, a build-up of lipids in the blood occurs.

Factors which may contribute to producing this effect include:

- Deliberate dieting of fat ponies, e.g. starvation of laminitic ponies.
- Pregnancy in small ponies, particularly Shetlands.
- Lactation.
- Energy starvation arising from illness.
- Heavy worm burden.
- Transportation stress increases cortisol levels, which can make the animal susceptible.

Signs

- Loss of appetite.
- Depression and weakness.
- Rapid loss of condition.
- Colic signs as the horse experiences abdominal pain because of swelling of the liver.
- The animal may stand over the water trough 'playing' with water without drinking.
- Breathing difficulties.
- Initially constipation followed by a greasy, fatty diarrhoea.
- Heavily pregnant mares may abort or foal early.
- Lactating mares may stop producing milk.

Treatment

1. Adequate food usually corrects the condition if diagnosed very early.
2. The vet may prescribe insulin and glucose.
3. Heparin may be prescribed as it increases the rate of fat removal from the blood.

Between 60 and 70 per cent of cases do not recover.

ITQ 66 What is hyperlipaemia?

LYMPHANGITIS

Lymphangitis is inflammation of the lymph vessels. The lymphatic system plays an important role in the maintenance of the balance between water in the bloodstream and in the tissue spaces between the cells. This balance depends upon the correct concentration of salts and proteins in the bloodstream. Any factor that upsets this can affect the lymphatic system's efficiency.

Causes

This condition can be caused by infection (e.g. as a result of a wound), or through dietary imbalance. In the case of dietary imbalance, excess feeding and too little exercise disturbs the protein:electrolyte balance with the result that the lymphatic system is unable to carry away waste material and excess fluid.

Some individuals are prone to recurrent bouts of lymphangitis for no obvious reason and once a horse has suffered from lymphangitis the condition is likely to recur.

Signs

- Inflamed hind leg – often the entire leg up to the stifle is hot and swollen. The lymph nodes can sometimes be seen prominently on the inside of the limb.
- The horse will be in great pain and reluctant to bear weight on the affected limb.
- Serum may exude through the skin and the lymph nodes will be enlarged.
- The horse may sweat and tremble.
- Loss of appetite.
- Fever.
- Often the limb will remain thickened.

Treatment

1. The vet will administer antibiotics to tackle any infection.
2. Non-steroidal anti-inflammatory drugs (e.g. phenylbutazone) will be administered to relieve the swelling.
3. Diuretics will increase fluid excretion.
4. The diet must be adjusted immediately – reduce all high protein and carbohydrate feeds and give only low-energy feeds and hay.
5. Cold treatments and bandaging will reduce swelling, as will controlled walking exercise.

DEHYDRATION

Dehydration means, essentially, loss of water, and that lies at the heart of the condition. The normal range of bodily water content of healthy horses is 50–70 per cent by weight. The average is 60 per cent; in young horses, about 70 per cent. However, the impact of dehydration goes far beyond the simple loss of water; fundamental metabolic processes are compromised and severe cases can lead to death. The following points are key to an understanding of the condition.

Primary water loss (true or pure dehydration) is caused when water intake is inadequate, normally because the horse cannot drink, e.g. as a result of neglect or a disease which causes difficulty in swallowing, such as tetanus.

In many cases, however, the loss is not of pure water, but of water-based fluids and **electrolytes**, and this will disturb metabolic functions. Normal metabolism and cellular functions can only continue in the presence of the correct balance of fluids and electrolytes. Electrolytes are substances that conduct electricity through their **ions**. Ions are atoms with either a positive electrical charge (a **cation**) or a negative electrical charge (an **anion**). There must be a balance between anions and cations to ensure electrical neutrality and therefore normal cell function.

The most important electrolytes in equine metabolism are sodium chloride (common salt), potassium, calcium, magnesium, phosphorus and the trace elements iron, copper, zinc, cobalt, selenium, sulphur and iodine. If these substances, and the requisite volumes of fluid, are lost from the body and not replaced, there will be disturbance of the metabolic processes at a cellular level.

A loss of up to 5 per cent of body fluids will result in mild dehydration, 8 per cent moderate dehydration, 10 per cent is severe and fluid loss of 12–15 per cent is life-threatening.

ITQ 67 What are the following?

a. Electrolyte.

b. Ion.

c. Cation.

d. Anion.

Causes

Dehydration can be induced by certain factors in an otherwise healthy horse, or it can be a consequence of disease.

IN THE HEALTHY HORSE

- In a working horse this condition generally occurs as a result of excessive sweating by a horse who does not receive enough to drink. This can happen, for example, at an event or competition, especially one in which the horse is required to undertake considerable exertion. At such times, horses should be offered water very frequently (every 45 minutes, or more frequently in hot weather).

- It can simply be the result of poor stable management/neglect – the horse being left without water for several hours.

- Lack of water during transportation. Many modes of transport do not have particularly good ventilation and because of this, and stress induced by travelling, horses may sweat during transit. All horses, including those who have not sweated, should be offered water frequently (at least every $1^1/_2$ hours on a long journey; more frequently in hot weather). Wherever possible a water bucket should be secured in a position allowing the horse free access to water during the journey.

IN THE SICK HORSE

- Haemorrhage
- Diarrhoea.
- Shock.

- Accumulation of fluid in the bowel, e.g. resulting from an obstruction (see Colic, this chapter).

In diarrhoea or intestinal obstruction, large volumes of fluid (water and electrolytes) may be lost into the bowel lumen. This form of fluid loss is particularly dangerous as sodium is the major solute responsible for maintenance of plasma osmotic pressure and circulating volume. When the horse suffers from diarrhoea, bicarbonate is also lost, which disrupts the acid-base balance.

In the case of an obstruction, normal secretions enter the intestine and cannot reach the lower part of the tract where they would normally be resorbed. In addition, within 12 hours of obstruction, the bowel mucosa (mucus-secreting cells) begin to secrete rather than absorb fluids and electrolytes. These fluid losses are borne by the extra cellular fluid which is drawn from the blood vessels and tissue spaces. The blood volume becomes reduced – the blood becomes more concentrated and has a thicker consistency.

The reduced blood flow leads to oxygen starvation within the tissues, causing the cells to switch to anaerobic metabolism. This leads to a build-up of lactic acid which disrupts the pH levels in the cells. The cells become acidotic and normal function is impaired.

Acidity is measured on the pH scale which ranges from 1–14. A pH of 7 is 'neutral'. Solutions with a pH of less than 7 are **acids**; those with a pH greater than 7 are **alkalis** or **bases**. For cells to function normally plasma must have a pH of 7.35–7.45. Any deviation from this will affect cellular and enzyme function.

When the plasma pH falls the horse is referred to as **acidotic**. Accumulated endotoxins may then be absorbed, resulting in further deterioration of the circulatory system.

ITQ 68 Give four causes of dehydration in the horse.

1.

2.

3.

4.

ITQ 69

a. What is the optimum pH of plasma?

b. What causes the horse to become acidotic?

Signs

The horse appears dull and lethargic.
- Dry skin loses its pliability (see skin pinch test, next page).

- Capillary and jugular refill times increase (See capillary and jugular refill tests below).
- Eyeballs recede into their sockets. This is especially noticeable in dehydrated foals.
- Weight loss.
- Small, dry faeces.
- Decreased urine.
- Acidosis (blood becomes acidic).
- Weakened pulse.
- In extreme cases the horse may go into a coma before death occurs.

Testing for Dehydration

The following tests can be used to assess whether a horse is dehydrated, and to give an indication of the extent of the condition.

The skin pinch test. Dehydration causes a loss of skin elasticity – normally a pinch of skin from the neck would recoil to its usual position immediately. If the skin remains 'tented', taking longer than 2 seconds to recoil, the horse is dehydrated. The longer it takes to recoil, the more dehydrated the horse. A recoil time of 4 seconds or more indicates serious dehydration.

The capillary refill test. Pressure on the horse's gum will press the blood out of the capillaries, causing the area to blanch. Normally the blanched area will return to pink as soon as the pressure is removed, as the blood flows back through the capillaries. If this takes 2 seconds or more, it indicates that the blood is too thick to circulate easily through the capillary network. A refill time of 4 seconds or more indicates a very serious (life-threatening) problem.

The jugular refill test. The blood can be squeezed from the jugular vein by running the thumb or forefinger down the jugular groove. When empty, you can feel the collapsed vein refill and become distended with blood. Normally this would happen immediately. If it takes longer than 2 seconds this can be considered a warning sign. As with the other tests, a refill time of 4 seconds or more indicates a life-threatening degree of dehydration.

Haematology. The blood can be tested to determine the degree of dehydration.
- The proportion of red blood cells to plasma is measured as a percentage; this measurement is known as the **packed cell volume** (**PCV**). The normal range of PCV is between 35 and 50 per cent; the average is 40 per cent. When a horse is dehydrated the PCV increases. A PCV of 55 per cent is very serious, 60 per cent + is grave, 65 per cent + is probably terminal.

- **Plasma proteins**. This reading is taken in conjunction with PCV at regular intervals to monitor the horse's progress.

- **Serum chloride levels**. If these are low this indicates electrolyte loss.
- **Blood pH and lactate levels**. These help to ascertain the degree of acidosis.

Treatment

Depending on the cause and extent of the dehydration, fluid therapy may be either immediately life-saving or supportive.

1. The simplest way for a horse to take in more fluid is to drink water. Depending on the nature of the dehydration, the horse should be offered plain water and an electrolyte solution. However, horses who are unused to electrolytes may not like the taste and refuse to drink the solution.

2. Paste electrolytes in wormer-type syringes can be given orally. These are used to good effect during endurance rides. Dosage instructions must be followed carefully and water must be offered.

3. If a stomach tube can be passed and the intestine is normal, water may be given 'orally'. This must be done at a steady rate, never hurriedly.

4. The sick horse will probably not want to drink and, if dehydrated, will need fluids administered intravenously. **Intravenous infusion** is the method of choice for effective fluid therapy as it ensures the fluid enters the circulatory system immediately. In aseptic conditions, an indwelling catheter over a needle is inserted into one of the jugular veins on the neck. Once the catheter is in place the needle is fully withdrawn and a three-way stopcock placed on the end. It is then sutured to the skin to prevent movement. The fluid administration set is suspended above the horse and attached to the catheter via a flexible coiled line. The fluid will drip through at a rate calculated by the vet or veterinary nurse according to the horse's bodyweight and level of dehydration.

5. *To correct acidosis.* The degree of acidosis must be ascertained – this is normally done through pH and blood gas analysis. Sodium bicarbonate is infused.

Prevention

The following measures will help prevent healthy horses becoming dehydrated.
- Ensure that horses always have access to fresh, clean water.
- During endurance rides allow the horse to drink frequently.
- Offer water to horses during transit and whilst at events. In hot conditions this must be done frequently.
- Add electrolytes to the feed or administer orally before and after a long journey or competition.

DISORDERS OF THE GASTROINTESTINAL TRACT
COLIC

Colic is not a specific disease; it is the term used to describe the clinical manifestation of abdominal pain. According to the specifics, a case of colic will be termed either **medical** or **surgical**. Colic varies in severity from a mild transient form to a much more serious form where the blood supply to the gut is compromised. The latter type is life-threatening and requires immediate surgery to save the horse. *It is very important that the vet is called for all colic cases.*

Medical Colics

There are four main types of medical colics, most of which respond to prompt veterinary treatment.

Spasmodic colic is the most common form of colic. It occurs as a result of localized spasms of the muscles of the small intestine which disrupts normal peristalsis, causing intermittent painful episodes.

Gastric colic occurs as a result of over-distension of the stomach. This may be caused by a build-up of gas, e.g. after eating grass cuttings or excessive numbers of apples which ferment in the stomach, or after eating unsoaked sugar beet pulp, which then expands within the stomach.

Flatulent or tympanitic colic occurs as a result of excessive accumulation of gas from fermented food, which leads to distension of the intestines (tympany). The abdomen may be visibly distended. Because of the tympany, the large intestine becomes very unstable and is prone to twisting.

Impacted or obstructed colic occurs when food matter, hay or straw accumulates (impacts), often at the **pelvic flexure** of the large colon. This is the narrowest part of the large colon where the gut turns back on itself through 180 degrees.

Any interference with the passage of intestinal contents constitutes an obstruction. If the obstruction is not diagnosed and treated it can lead to damage to the gut wall. If severe, this may lead to endotoxic shock, which is potentially life-threatening.

OBSTRUCTIONS

Impacted or obstructed colic occurs in two main forms:

Simple obstructions are those whereby there is no compromise to the blood supply. An example of this would be a large colon impaction (constipation). The muscular waves of the intestines increase initially, becoming spasmodic and adding to the discomfort already felt. Large quantities of fluids; saliva, gastric, pancreatic and biliary secretions accumulate in the upper digestive tract, unable to pass the obstruction to reach the lower, absorbent surfaces.

As the intestine becomes distended, more fluid is drawn in from the circulatory system and, as pressure builds up, pain increases. These secretions may remain within the tract, unable to be resorbed into the system, or they may be expelled nasally.

Body salts and electrolytes are also lost in the fluid. This loss of body fluids from the system causes a reduction in cardiac output and central venous pressure; the horse will then be in a state of shock.

The site of the impaction will affect the pain felt by the horse – if low in the bowel it will show as a dull pain, less severe and protracted. The closer the impaction is to the anus, the easier it is for the vet to reach. A high obstruction, e.g. at the ileo-caecal junction, will cause greater pain and be out of reach.

Strangulating obstructions are those whereby the blood supply is compromised. A 'medical' obstructed colic can become a surgical case if, for example, it results in a length of gut twisting over on itself.

Surgical Colics

The blood supply may be obstructed (strangulated) as a result of one of the following.

Twisted gut (**torsion**). The intestinal tract may have twisted over on itself. This is the most serious form of obstruction as the blood supply to the twisted portion is immediately lost.

Bowel malposition. Part of the intestinal tract may become trapped in an abnormal position.

Intussusception. A length of the intestine may pass into the length lying just beyond it, rather like a telescope closing up. This is most common in foals and yearlings and is often caused by ascarid burden or redworm damage.

Hernia (**umbilical or inguinal**). A loop of gut passes into the hernia sac and becomes trapped as a result of swelling and engorgement of the gut wall. The lack of blood supply, and therefore of oxygen, to the gut wall causes degeneration of the tissue and allows leakage of bacterial toxins into the abdominal cavity. The toxins are absorbed through the lining of the cavity (peritoneum) into the bloodstream, causing the first stages of endotoxic (septic) shock.

Pedunculated lipoma. This is a benign fatty tumour attached to the mesentery by string-like lengths of tissue. These can wind around the small intestine, blocking the passage of food and compromising the blood supply. Lipomas tend to occur in older horses.

THE EFFECTS OF A STRANGULATING OBSTRUCTION

Initially, in cases of strangulating obstruction, arterial blood at a higher pressure pumps into the strangulated part, but venous outflow is obstructed. Blood pressure drops then the venous return of blood to the heart becomes diminished.

The severe drop in blood pressure stimulates the secretion of vasoactive chemicals which then cause the blood vessels to constrict. The constriction of the arterioles and venules leads to a further reduced blood flow, resulting in the pooling of blood in the body tissue.

When tissue is deprived of its blood supply and dies, this is referred to as **infarction**. Infarction leads to the production of bacterial toxins. Any leaking toxins have a direct effect on the walls of small blood vessels, allowing the escape of blood proteins. This further reduces blood pressure as fluid escapes and pools in the tissues. This situation is called endotoxic shock.

Pooling results in oxygen starvation within the tissues, causing the cells to switch to anaerobic metabolism. This leads to a great disruption of the pH levels in the cells with a very marked build-up of lactic acid. Death follows within a few hours.

ITQ 70 Name the four types of medical colic and describe each briefly.

1.

2.

3.

4.

ITQ 71 What is the 'pelvic flexure' and why is it significant in impacted colics?

ITQ 72 The intestines become distended with fluid when an impaction is present.

a. What are these fluids?

b. What happens if this situation is not corrected?

ITQ 73
a. What causes the blood pressure to drop in cases of strangulating obstruction?

b. What is infarction?

c. Why does infarction contribute to the further reduction in blood pressure?

d. Why is there an increase in the amount of lactic acid within the cells?

Causes

CAUSES OF SPASMODIC COLIC

- Irregular feeding routine.
- A sudden change in diet.
- Nervous, anxious types are more prone.
- Exercising hard too soon after a feed – always allow 1^1/$_2$ hours.
- Unusual physical activity.
- Taking a long, cold drink either after eating a feed or whilst very hot and sweating.
- Fatigue.
- Stress – this can be as a result of competing, or a long journey.
- Damage caused by migrating redworm larvae (sometimes referred to as **verminous colic**).

CAUSES OF GASTRIC COLIC

- Gorging on large quantities of food, e.g. after getting into the feed room.
- Eating too many green apples, e.g. access to an orchard.
- Eating lawn mowings – this is *very* dangerous as mowings are highly fermentative in the horse's gut.
- Eating unsoaked sugar beet nuts.

CAUSES OF TYMPANITIC COLIC

- Eating lawn mowings.
- Greedy feeding on new grass or clover, particularly in spring.
- Sudden change in concentrates.
- Mouldy feed or hay/haylage (fermentation may have started in the bag/bale).
- Eating poisonous plants such as ragwort or acorns – the horse may show signs of colic as well as signs of poisoning.

CAUSES OF IMPACTED COLIC

- Poor worming regime. Strongyle infestation can cause partial or complete obstruction of the gut. Migrating large strongyle larvae also cause damage to the lining of the main artery supplying the gut. Blood clots break away from the lining and obstruct the blood vessels supplying the gut. The reduced blood supply can interrupt normal peristalsis, causing a mild, transient colic. If, however, the blood supply is reduced to the point that tissue death (infarction) occurs, surgery will be needed to remove the affected portion of gut.
- Sand colic results from grazing on sandy soil and, less commonly, from drinking from a stream with a sandy bed. Sand colic is particularly dangerous, often proving fatal.
- Eating dry bran or unsoaked sugar beet pulp.
- Eating straw bedding.
- Poor quality, coarse hay.
- Faulty dentition, causing failure to chew food properly.
- Sudden enforced rest, e.g. when a horse is on box rest because of lameness or bad winter weather. The lack of normal movement and the stress of confinement can trigger colic in certain horses.

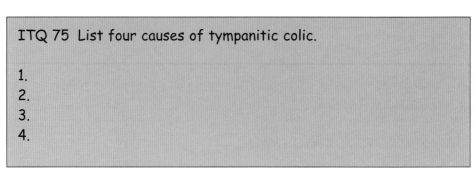

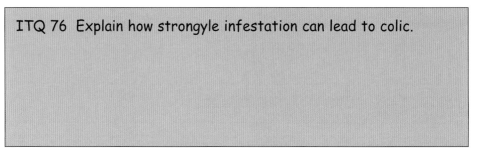

ITQ 76 Explain how strongyle infestation can lead to colic.

Signs

Although they may give some indication of the type of colic occurring, early signs of colic often relate to the levels of discomfort rather than the specific form.

Early signs of mild abdominal pain shown by the horse may include:
- Disinterest in food or water.
- Quiet, lethargic attitude.
- Passing fewer droppings than normal.
- Pawing at the ground, looking around at his flanks.
- Appearing to be in discomfort.
- Grinding teeth/yawning.

In the early stages of an impacted colic the horse may:
- Walk backwards into the corner of the stable.
- Lie flat out in the stable. He will not rise and may make groaning sounds.
- Appear to be trying to urinate.
- Adopt a position similar to a sitting dog.

If the pain is more severe the horse may:
- Sweat – generally or in patches.
- Repeatedly attempt to lie down and roll. Spasmodic colics tend to cause rolling as the pain increases.

- Pace around the stable.
- If the pain is very severe the horse may 'throw himself down' onto the ground, as opposed to getting down to roll.

ITQ 77 List the early signs of mild abdominal pain.

1.

2.

3.

4.

5.

Immediate Action

- Call the vet if the horse shows mild colic signs that do not pass after 10 minutes, or immediately if the signs are more serious, e.g. sweating and rolling.

- If the horse is lying quietly, it is not necessary to make him walk around whilst waiting for the vet to arrive. Make sure the stable is well bedded down to prevent injury. Remove the water buckets and haynet to prevent injury if the horse rolls.

- In cold weather keep the horse comfortably warm. The type of rug used will depend on the weather and whether or not the horse has sweated. A thermal 'cooler' type of rug will wick sweat away from the coat, helping to keep him dry and prevent chilling.

- If the horse rolls violently and continually in the stable there is a danger that he will become cast and injure himself. If possible, lead him to a field or manège, keeping well away from hazards such as the fence, jumps, ditches, etc.

- A few minutes walking *may* stop the horse from rolling if the pain is not too severe but do not tire him by walking excessively.

The Veterinary Examination
AIMS

There are two main aims of the veterinary examination:

1. To establish that the horse really has colic. There are certain conditions which mimic colic – these are referred to as 'false' colics. The more common false colics include:
— Parturition.
— Uterine rupture.
— Retained placenta.
— Meconium retention in foals.

— Ruptured bladder.
— Pleurisy.
— EER.
— Laminitis.
— Scrotal hernia.

2. To establish the cause of the abdominal pain, i.e. to find out if the condition is mild and uncomplicated or potentially life-threatening.

ITQ 78

a. What is a 'false' colic?

b. Give three examples of 'false' colics.

1.

2.

3.

APPROACH TO DIAGNOSIS

The vet will follow a number of steps as necessary to reach a diagnosis.

1. **History**. The vet will need to know:
— The horse's age and breed.
— The duration of clinical signs – when was the horse actually last seen to be normal?
— The nature of the pain.
— The frequency of painful episodes.
— Faeces and urine – nature, quantity, when passed.
— Feeding regime.
— Worming regime.
— Exercise and workload.
— Existence of stable 'vices', e.g. wind-sucking.
— Previous medical history.

2. **Pain relief**. Whilst finding out the above information, the vet will watch the horse to ascertain the nature and severity of the pain. Once the horse's behavioural pattern has been noted the vet may decide to administer analgesics at that point, especially if the horse is distressed because of severe pain.

3. **Assessment of relevant criteria**. Table 2 shows the criteria assessed by the vet when an initial examination is made.

CRITERIA	GREEN Healthy responses	AMBER Warning signs – with prompt veterinary attention the horse has every chance of recovery	RED Danger signs – the prognosis is grave
Pulse rate (bpm) and character	25–40 regular	Rises sharply to 0–60 during spasms of pain, returning to normal as soon as pain ceases	60–80, which stays high during analgesia 80+ Weakened pulse
Pain	Absent	Intermittent (spasms) interspersed with pain-free periods	Continuously in severe pain
Mucous membranes	Salmon pink and moist	Pale and tacky	Brick-red conjunctival membranes, dry, bluish purple or greyish white lips
Eyes	Bright, clear	Glassy	Fixed stare Sunken eyeball
Capillary refill time	0–2 seconds	2–3 seconds	4+ seconds
Gut sounds	Normal	Reduced Increased	Absent
Respiratory rate	Relaxed Regular	Panting	Rapid, jerky Sighing
Faecal passage	Normal	Small, hard, dry faeces Diarrhoea	Absent (Faeces may be passed from the bowel behind an obstruction for up to 8–10 hours after obstruction)

Table 2 Assessing criteria in the horse with colic

4. **Rectal examination**. The abdomen can be examined per rectum and much useful information gained. The vet inserts a gloved, lubricated arm into the horse's rectum and feels for:

- Droppings in the rectum. These are removed and examined for strongyles, mucus, blood or shreds of mucous membranes.
- Absence of droppings. This may indicate an obstruction higher in the gut.
- Gaseous distension, indicating tympanitic colic.
- A dry rectal wall, possibly indicating grass sickness.
- Tight constriction of the rectum, which may indicate intestinal torsion (twisted gut).
- Pelvic flexure impaction.
- Gaseous distension of the pelvic flexure, which could indicate displacement or torsion of the colon.

5. **Nasogastric intubation (passing a stomach tube)**. The horse may need to be sedated and/or administered analgesics to make this procedure less difficult. The vet passes a flexible tube up the nostril, into the pharynx and, when the horse swallows, pushes it down the oesophagus and into the stomach.

This may aid diagnosis. For example, gas may escape from the stomach via the tube, indicating tympanitic colic. The release of gas will also relieve the pain.

The presence of large quantities of fluid and gas in the stomach may also be indicative of an obstruction in the small intestine.

In certain conditions, treatments such as fluids and/or liquid paraffin can be administered via the stomach tube. (This is not performed in cases where an obstruction is causing a build-up of fluids in the stomach.)

6. **Abdominal paracentesis (peritoneal tap)**. To aid assessment of the abdomen, a small sample of fluid is collected from the horse's abdominal cavity. The vet will clip and scrub the lowest part of the horse's abdomen and insert a needle to collect the fluid sample.

Normal peritoneal fluid is a clear pale straw colour. Where peritonitis (infection of the abdomen) is present the fluid will be cloudy. If the gut is ruptured the fluid will be a brownish colour, possibly containing food matter.

7. **Blood tests**. Laboratory investigation can provide an accurate picture of the horse's health status. Parameters to be monitored include:

- **Packed cell volume** (PCV). The percentage volume of red blood cells to whole blood is measured. The normal range is 35–50 per cent. When a horse is in shock the PCV increases. A PCV of 55 per cent is very serious, 60 per cent + is grave, 65 per cent + is probably terminal.
- **Serum chloride levels**. If these are low it indicates electrolyte loss.
- **Blood pH and lactate levels**. This helps to ascertain the degree of acidosis.

ITQ 79

a. What is the purpose of the rectal examination?

b. Give three examples of problems that may be identified through rectal examination.

1.

2.

3.

ITQ 80

a. What is the purpose of abdominal paracentesis?

b. Give another name for this procedure.

c. How is it performed?

ITQ 81 What information can be gained from a blood test?

Treatment

Depending on the diagnosis, treatment is likely to include one or more of the following.

Spasmolytic drugs. Buscopan (dipyrone) is the most commonly used antispasmodic drug. By reducing the muscle spasm, pain is relieved and often, in spasmodic colics, this is all that is needed. It is administered by intramuscular or intravenous injection.

Analgesia. Finadyne (flunixin meglumine) is a very effective non-steroidal anti-inflammatory drug with antipyretic (fever-reducing), antiendotoxic and analgesic qualities. In endotoxic cases, it may be administered along with antibiotics and plasma. However, the drug is so effective that it can be misleading, occasionally masking the pain and signs of deterioration of a serious colic. **Torbugesic** (butorphanol) acts on the central nervous system and produces an effective level of analgesia.

Sedatives. **Xylazine** provides potent analgesia and muscle relaxation. Sedation may be needed to allow rectal examination. **Domosedan** (detomidine) is another type of sedative, sometimes used in combination with Torbugesic.

Liquid paraffin may be administered (sometimes with saline solution) via the stomach tube to lubricate the gut and aid the passage of an impaction.

Decompression. Necessary in gastric and tympanitic colics, this involves relieving gastric tympany by nasogastric intubation. Walking sometimes helps to disperse the gaseous build-up.

Fluid therapy may be necessary to maintain body water, electrolyte and pH balance. This can be administered via the stomach tube or intravenously via a drip.

Hospitalization. If the vet suspects that the colic is complicated a recommendation will be made that the horse is admitted to the local veterinary hospital in case surgery is needed.

ITQ 82 What are the following?

a. Buscopan.

b. Finadyne.

c. Xylazine.

d. Torbugesic.

ITQ 83 How might the vet relieve gaseous distension in the stomach?

SURGERY

When a surgical colic is diagnosed a decision has to be made quickly as to whether surgery or euthanasia is to be performed. Factors which affect this decision include:

Prognosis. If the horse has been in shock for some time he is unlikely to benefit from surgery.

Distance to the nearest equine hospital/surgery. If the horse is in severe pain it would be traumatic to transport him a long distance.

Age. The older the horse, the less likely he is to recover from the trauma of surgery.

Cost. At the time of writing, colic surgery in Great Britain will cost in the region of £2,500–£4,000. Obviously the more complicated the case is, and the more veterinary attention, drugs, etc. that are needed, the more it will cost. It is easier to make a decision based on finance if you know that the horse is insured for this type of surgery.

> ITQ 84 When a surgical colic is diagnosed, what factors must be considered when deciding if surgery or euthanasia should be performed?

Aftercare
MEDICAL COLICS

In the case of medical colics which respond to treatment, once the vet has left, keep a close eye on the horse and only offer him a small, warm bran mash to eat. Replace wet rugs with dry ones and towel-dry any wet sweat patches to prevent him from catching a chill. Follow the vet's advice carefully and, if the horse's condition worsens, call the vet again.

POST-SURGERY

If colic surgery is carried out successfully, the horse will remain in the hospital until the vets deem him fit enough to return home. The vets will provide full and detailed written instructions on the aftercare of the horse once home. The aftercare will include attention to the following points.

- Restrict exercise. Box rest will be necessary initially. Gentle walking in hand will help to control swelling of the wound.

- Whilst the horse is on box rest, apply support bandages to the limbs to prevent filling.

- Provide inedible bedding. As the horse is to be confined for long periods he is likely to eat straw bedding. This could lead to an impaction.

- Check the wound two or three times a day. If it is discharging, tell the vet. Keep the wound clean with a Hibiscrub or Pevidine solution.

- Once the horse can be turned out, do so initially in a *very* small paddock. The horse should not be allowed to canter until at least three months after surgery.

- The vet will remove the sutures or staples about two weeks after surgery, by which time the skin will have healed but the underlying layers of muscle will still be weakened. (Hence restricted exercise.)

- Feed only easily digested non-heating concentrates mixed with warm, moist bran to keep the droppings soft. Feed soft, dampened hay and ensure a constant supply of clean, fresh water.

- Keep the horse warm in cold weather with lightweight rugs. A large area of the coat will have been clipped prior to surgery and the horse may have lost weight during the post-operative period.

- Intestinal adhesions often occur after colic surgery, rendering the horse susceptible to further bouts of abdominal pain. Any signs of post-operative colic must be reported to the vet immediately.

ITQ 85 Why must the horse be box-rested initially after colic surgery?

ITQ 86 What complications may arise after colic surgery?

Prevention

Even with the best care, it is not always possible to eradicate the risk of colic. However, since it is potentially such a dangerous condition, all practical steps should be taken to try to avoid it. These include the following:

- Worm horses regularly.
- Have horses' teeth checked and rasped at least once a year.
- Introduce changes to the diet slowly.
- Feed only good quality feedstuffs.
- Allow $1^1/_2$ hours between feeding and exercising.
- Restrict access to new spring grass.
- Be sure that well-meaning neighbours don't feed garden waste, e.g. lawn mowings, hedge clippings to horses.
- Use inedible bedding.
- Where sand colic is a risk, ispaghula husk (**Isogel** and **Fybogel**) can be used to good effect. This is a powder that is added to a feed and well dampened. When wet it forms a jelly-like consistency which, once eaten, helps to bind any ingested sand into a bolus. As the sand is kept in suspension it can pass through the gut. These powders should be used according to the vet's instructions. They are generally recommended for

use once a week in winter, when grazing is poor and horses are inclined to pull at the root mat. Summer use is dictated by the quality of the grazing – if grazing is good, horses are less likely to graze right down to the root mat and are therefore less likely to ingest sand. (If the risk of sand colic is significant, alternative grazing should be considered. Also, in winter, providing piles of hay will make it less likely that horses will graze on the root mat.)

- The risk of colic arising on long journeys may be reduced prior to transit, by feeding probiotics. Probiotics boost the gut's microbe population, which promotes healthy gut function.

> **ITQ 87 What can be done to reduce the incidence of sand colic in horses grazing regularly on sandy soils?**

GRASS SICKNESS

Also referred to as **equine dysautonomia**, grass sickness is a disease of horses, ponies and donkeys whereby degeneration of the autonomic nerves controlling gut function causes paralysis of the gut.

It occurs virtually exclusively in equids with access to grass and until recently had a mortality rate approaching 100 per cent. Thanks to advances in treatment, the recovery rate has improved in animals suffering from the chronic form.

Cause

Grass sickness seems to occur more commonly in animals aged between 3 and 7 years with peak incidence from April to July. It is associated with spells of fine and dry weather. However, the exact cause is unknown – much research is being undertaken and one theory is that a fungal toxin acquired from pasture may be involved. As it is impossible to perform a biopsy on the affected group of nerves, confirmation of the diagnosis can only be made after the horse has died.

Signs and Types

There appear to be three basic types of the disease. Since the signs (especially of the acute and sub-acute forms) include intestinal discomfort, they may be confused with simple – albeit severe – colic. This is another reason why 'coliky' symptoms should always be referred to the vet: veterinary diagnosis will differentiate between colic and grass sickness.

Acute. The symptoms are severe – the horse shows acute pain, sweating, rolling, looking round at the flanks and pawing at the ground. Because of paralysis of the oesophagus the horse is unable to swallow, so drools. Fluid that cannot be moved on accumulates in the stomach, causing distension, and gastric contents may reflux out of the nostrils. Rupture of the stomach may occur.

The large intestine becomes impacted, causing constipation. If any droppings are passed, the pellets are small, hard and may have a 'cheesy' coating of mucus. The horse may have muscle tremors and areas of patchy sweating. Acute grass sickness remains invariably fatal and, once the diagnosis has been made, euthanasia is generally performed.

Subacute. The signs are similar to those of the acute form, but are less severe. Complete paralysis of the gut does not occur, thus allowing small quantities of food to be consumed. The horse will, however, show some difficulty in swallowing, moderate signs of colic, muscle tremors and rapid weight loss and will either die, need to be euthanased or, in some cases, the condition passes into the chronic stage.

Chronic. The signs tend to develop more slowly. There may or may not be signs of colic. Loss of appetite and varying degrees of difficulty in swallowing are followed by severe weight loss.

Approximately 30 per cent of these cases make a complete recovery.

Treatment

Treatment is not currently considered in acute and many subacute cases.

Chronic cases may be treated if they are not in pain and still have an interest in life. Treatment involves the use of drugs to increase gut activity, keeping the horse warm and feeding highly nutritious, easily swallowed mashes. Successful treatment takes several months, but eventual recovery is complete.

ENTERITIS

This term describes inflammation of the small intestines, accompanied by diarrhoea. The condition is included in this chapter on Non-infectious Diseases because, although the causal agent *may* be bacterial, there are various other causes.

Causes

Any agents, such as bacteria, fungi, antibiotics or excess protein, which disturb the natural flora in the intestine. Some agents, such as the salmonella bacteria, erode the intestinal villi.

Treatment

The primary cause must be identified and treated.

Enteritis can be fatal, especially in foals – very careful management is needed to prevent dehydration. If necessary, a blood sample will be taken to assess the degree of dehydration and the vet will administer fluid therapy via an intravenous drip.

CHAPTER SUMMARY

This chapter has covered some of the most frequently seen non-infectious diseases of the horse, some of which have the potential to be very serious. Colic, for example, can range from mild abdominal discomfort to a life-threatening condition and, unfortunately, even mild colics can deteriorate quickly if not treated promptly. Dehydration, too, can be vastly more significant than the horse 'needing a drink'; in its most serious forms it, like colic, can be life-threatening. Knowledge of these diseases and good management can help prevent them from occurring in the first place. These attributes are also useful in helping to prevent the onset of some cases of conditions to which many horses are inherently susceptible, such as exertional rhabdomyolysis.

CHAPTER 6

LAMENESS

The aims and objectives of this chapter are to explain:

- The procedure for examining the lame horse.
- The diagnostic aids and techniques used by the vet.
- The signs, causes and treatment of a range of ailments and disorders that can cause lameness.
- The need for correct rehabilitation.

Lameness is a disturbance of the horse's natural gait, normally associated with pain and is a sign that disease or injury is present. Examination of the horse is necessary to find out which leg he is lame on and the nature of the disease or injury.

It is necessary to be able to differentiate between lameness, as caused by disease or injury and a defective gait, as caused by faulty conformation or stiffness (arising from age or fatigue).

EXAMINATION TO DIAGNOSE LAMENESS

The initial examination may be divided into the following procedures:

- Reference to medical history and reported signs.

- Observation at rest.

- Observation during movement.

- Palpation of the limbs.

- Passive movement of the joints.

- Checking the spine (if necessary).

Examination may reveal the root cause of lameness – if not, it will at least provide information for the vet. If, after these initial procedures have been followed, the cause of the lameness has not become apparent, the vet will employ more sophisticated measures, such as nerve-blocking and X-rays, to detect the problem. Let us examine how to follow these diagnostic procedures in more detail.

MEDICAL HISTORY AND REPORTED SIGNS

The first point to consider is whether there is a relevant history of illness or lameness. Also, has the horse recently slipped badly or fallen whilst jumping/working, or been kicked or cast in his box? Other background points to note are:

- Breeding and age.

- The purpose for which the horse is kept. If for competition, the type of competition and details of performance at these events.

- Whether the horse is stabled, grass-kept or a combination of both.

- Diet. Any vitamin or mineral supplements must be noted. Also, does the horse have a healthy appetite? (Inappetance may indicate other underlying problems.)

When the horse has been ridden, have there been signs of:

- Stiffness, resistance or evasion of the bit?

- A 'cold back' or excessive hollowing?

- Difficulty when going either up or down hill?

- Difficulty on corners and tight circles?

- An unwillingness to jump?

- A frequent change of leg at canter or gallop?

- The horse trying to bump the rider from one diagonal to another at rising trot?

Other pertinent questions include:

- When did the horse become lame/for how long has he been lame?

- Was the onset of lameness sudden and, if so, what was the horse doing at the time?

- Are there any swellings, soft or hard, that are normal or abnormal on the horse's limbs?

- Have any new signs of heat or swelling arisen since the lameness?

- Does the horse move evenly on either rein?

- Does the going make any difference? Is the lameness better or worse on hard or soft ground?

Once all these facts have been established, the observation can begin.

OBSERVATION AT REST

Without entering the stable, the horse's general stance should be observed, and reference made to the following points:

- Does he stand with the weight distributed evenly on all four legs? Resting a hind leg is no cause for concern, but resting or 'pointing' a foreleg is indicative of trouble.

- Does he shift his weight from one forefoot to another? This may be seen if pain is present in both forefeet, for example with laminitis. Also, does the horse lie down excessively?

- Has he dug up his bedding? Horses with pain in the heel region of the foot may stand with their heels raised on mounds of bedding.

- Note his overall condition as best as possible (bearing in mind that he may still be rugged up) – does he look disinterested or in pain?

Having put on a bridle, try to position the horse so that he is on a clear level surface, preferably not a bedded-down floor. Good light is essential if you are to examine the horse properly. Use a systematic approach, working upwards from the foot.

- Pick up the feet; pick them out and examine them. Note the wear of the shoes, if he is shod. Are the shoes a normal design or a remedial design? Has a shoe slipped or been lost? Is anything wedged in the shoe, e.g. a stone?

- Feel for heat in the hoof wall. Compare the hoof walls.

- Look at the pastern/foot axis of all four limbs – are the respective pairs similar?

- Look at the size and shape of the feet – are the respective pairs the same? One small, boxy foot could indicate a problem.

- Look for obvious signs such as bleeding, cuts, lumps, heat and swelling.

- Remove any rugs and note temperature, pulse and respiratory rates – any increases in rates may indicate pain and/or infection (NB: the individual horse's normal resting rates must be known for this to be of value.)

- Look at the muscular development on each side – it should be even. Note any lumps or sores on the spine. Look at the horse from behind – the hips should appear level.

Once you have made these observations you will need to see the horse moving. The exceptions to this would be a horse who has suffered obvious tendon/ligament breakdown, one who cannot bear weight on the lame leg, (i.e. is fracture lame), or if a fracture is suspected.

OBSERVATION DURING MOVEMENT

Usually, a hard and level surface is needed. However, lameness caused by soft tissue injuries often shows more clearly when the horse is lunged or trotted up on a soft surface.

- You must observe the horse from the front, back and side.

- Depending upon the degree of lameness, it may be apparent at walk. However, if the lameness is of a mild nature it is preferable to move the horse into trot straight away before the lameness 'walks off'.

- A steady trot on a loose rein will show up most types of lameness. However, if the horse is trotted too quickly this may actually disguise a problem. As well as being led on a straight line the horse should be lunged on a hard surface, as this often accentuates the effects of unsoundness.

- In addition to looking for lameness you can also *listen* for any irregularities in the hoof beats, although it is necessary for the horse to be either shod or unshod all round in order to hear a clear beat.

ITQ 88 When observing the horse in the stable, what two signs are indicative of problems in the limbs?

1.

2.

ITQ 89 Under what circumstances would you not trot up a lame horse?

Foreleg Lameness

- When the problem is in one leg only, the withers, neck and head appear to lower as the sound leg comes to the ground. As the unsound leg bears the weight, the horse raises his head in order to reduce weightbearing – this hoof beat may also sound lighter.

- If the horse is lame in both forelegs, the steps will be short and pottery and the action stilted, with decreased shoulder movement. If the lameness is fairly equal in each leg there may be no nodding of the head and the horse may appear to be 'going even'.

- If one leg is worse than the other a degree of head nodding is generally visible – but the less lame leg must not be overlooked. Nerve-blocking of the worse leg will show up the lameness in the other more noticeably.

Hind Leg Lameness

- As the lame hind leg comes to the ground, the croup will be raised and the step made lighter. The result of raising the croup is that the head and neck will be lowered. As the sound hind leg comes to the ground, so this is reversed – the croup lowers and the head and neck are raised.

- If both hind legs are unsound, the stride will be shortened and the action wobbly and/or straddling in manner. The horse may also find it difficult to step backwards.

- Watching the horse move from the side enables variations in stride length or reduced joint flexion to be observed.

- When the horse is turned, notice how he bears weight on the inside hind leg. Turning the horse tightly around on the spot may accentuate the effects of a hind leg problem.

PALPATION OF THE LIMBS

The suspect limb must now be examined carefully for signs of heat, swelling and/or pain.

- The foot should be picked out again and, if muddy, scrubbed. Ninety per cent of all lamenesses originate in the foot – it is therefore imperative that the foot is carefully examined first. A drawing knife should be used to scrape at the sole, allowing you to check the sole for bruising or puncture wounds.

- Assess the condition of the shoe, making a note of uneven wear and loose or missing nails.

- Feel the walls of each pair of hooves with the back of your hand and compare the temperature of each.

- Hoof testers may be used to apply pressure around the hoof. The horse will be likely to flinch if pain is felt. Sole pads will have to be removed before the hoof tester is used. Test the other hooves too – some sensitive horses flinch and react to the testers even when there is no pain in the foot, so you need to assess the validity of the horse's reaction.

- If lameness within the foot is suspected, it may be necessary to have the shoe removed and to look further for bruising, corns, puncture wounds or an abscess.

- If the cause of foot lameness is still not apparent the advice of the farrier and vet must be sought, as further investigation will be necessary determine which area within the foot is affected.

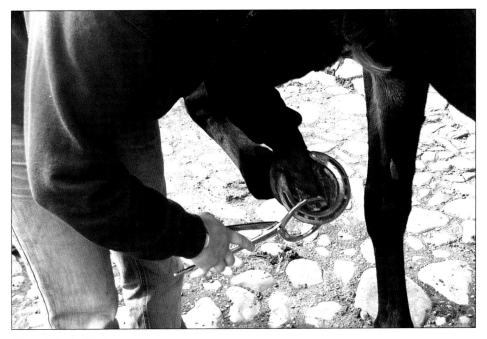

Figure 17 Hoof testers

- If the problem does not appear to be within the foot, continue the examination of the limb by feeling around the coronary band and heels. It is in this area, to the rear of the foot, that sidebones may be felt. Instead of being able to compress the coronet, a hard, bony lump may be felt. Also, feel the front of the pastern – a lump here could indicate the formation of a high ringbone.

- Next, continue to work up the pastern to the fetlock joint. Heat and swelling laterally may indicate damage to one or more of the ligaments of the joint, whilst inflammation at the rear of the joint could indicate sesamoiditis.

- Between the fetlock joint and the knee or hock, a careful examination must be made of the ligaments and tendons, feeling for heat and/or swelling, however slight.

- Heat and swelling may also be found on the inside of the limb, in the region of the splint bones.

- In the foreleg the knee, elbow and shoulder must be examined and, in the hind leg, the hock, stifle and hip.

- At all the above stages, compare the suspect limb to the sound one.

PASSIVE MOVEMENT OF THE JOINTS

In what is usually referred to as a **flexion test**, the individual joint is flexed manually to stress the ligaments and accentuate any problems. Note, however, that it is not possible to flex the hock without the stifle and vice versa.

The joint is flexed to the limit of its range and held in this position for approximately 1–2 minutes. The horse is then trotted on and any increase of lameness after the first three strides is noted. This test can be adapted for most of the joints of the horse.

- When trying to identify lameness in the shoulder, the foreleg should be extended as far forward as possible. The horse may well indicate pain by pulling backwards violently and handler safety must be considered.

- Stifle lameness may be shown by the horse keeping the stifle joint mostly flexed whether at rest or during movement.

- A problem in the hip may cause the toe to move outward instead of in straight alignment with the body. If pain is felt in the joints of the hind limb, the horse will seem to hold his leg up and keep weight off it whilst the flexion test is being carried out.

The joints may be extended, as opposed to flexed, by standing the horse on a wedge (toe up) for 1–2 minutes. Trotting on immediately may show up a more marked lameness in some instances.

Flexion tests are an aid to diagnosis but are not generally reliable enough to give a definite diagnosis. Most problems within a joint need to be confirmed with X-rays.

CHECKING THE SPINE

If it is suspected that the problem lies within the spine, it is possible to check whether the horse has a normal range of spinal movement. This is best done before exercise, to ensure that the muscles have not loosened up. The range of movement is as follows.

Ventroflexion (arching).
Dorsiflexion (hollowing).
Lateral flexion (sideways).

To test for ventroflexion, press a hand firmly beneath the abdomen just behind the girth line – this should result in the horse arching his spine. Running your fingers or a pen ventrally along the horse's abdomen also causes most horses to arch the spine.

The horse should hollow away from pressure applied either side of the withers, and running a hand firmly down the length of his back applying pressure either side of the spinal process should cause the horse to curve his body away in lateral flexion.

The horse should be capable of turning his neck so that he can touch his ribs with his muzzle on either side. Offer a carrot to encourage the horse to flex laterally.

The spine should also be checked for swellings and saddle sores.

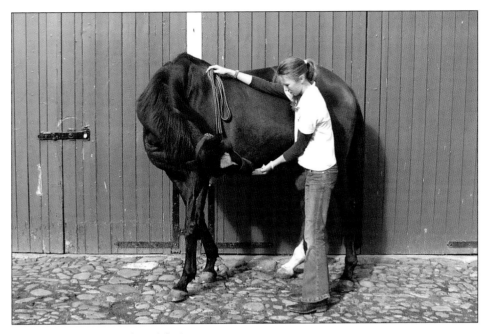

Figure 18 Encouraging lateral flexion

DIAGNOSTIC AIDS

In addition to the examination procedure described, the vet may use certain techniques to assist or confirm diagnosis.

NERVE-BLOCKING

The vet may block the nerves supplying the suspected area as an aid to a more accurate diagnosis. Local anaesthetic is injected into the area around the nerve, normally starting with the lower aspect of the limb. Assessing skin sensation in the area supplied by the nerve, by pressing with a pen or similar object, checks the effect of the block. Once the area is desensitized, the horse is trotted up. If the horse still appears lame, further anaesthetic may be injected higher up the limb. Once this has taken effect the horse may be trotted up again and, if he is sound, it may be deduced that the problem lies within that particular area.

Once the vet has identified the site of the problem as accurately as possible, imaging techniques can be used to produce pictures of deep structures of the horse's body. Imaging techniques include radiography, ultrasonography, scintigraphy and thermography.

RADIOGRAPHY

Radiographs (X-rays) are frequently needed in the diagnosis of lameness, especially if a fracture or bony change is suspected. However, changes that appear on a radiograph do not necessarily indicate the cause of the problem, and not all causes of lameness show radiographic changes. Therefore, radiographs should be used in conjunction with an accurate history and clinical examination of the problem area. Also, the vet may advocate taking radiographs of the sound limb for comparison.

In addition to diagnostic use, radiography is used following fracture surgery to monitor healing.

Explaining X-rays

X-rays are energy waves similar to light waves – members of the electromagnetic spectrum, as shown in Table 3. Waves of the electromagnetic spectrum have the following characteristics in common:

— They are produced by changing magnetic fields and changing electric fields.

— They are transverse waves with a range of frequencies and wavelengths.

— They all travel at the same speed, i.e. 300,000,000 metres per second.

— They do not need a material medium through which to travel.

The waves can be likened to the waves produced when a piece of rope moves up and down in an oscillating motion. The length of each complete oscillation is the **wavelength**. The **frequency** of the wave is the number of complete cycles per second, measured in Hertz (Hz).

		Radio waves	Micro- waves	Infra- red waves	Visible light	Ultra- violet waves	X-rays	Gamma rays	
Wavelength	Long	←							Short
Frequency	Low	→							High

Table 3 Summary of the waves of the electromagnetic spectrum

Electromagnetic radiation consists of energy in small 'packets' called **photons**. X-rays and gamma waves have high frequency, short wavelength and therefore high energy. X-rays, like the rest of the electromagnetic spectrum, have the following properties:

● They travel in straight lines.

● They interact with matter by being absorbed or scattered.

Additionally, X-rays can:

● Penetrate substances (because of their high energy) – and some may pass right through.

● Produce a hidden image on photographic film which can be made visible by processing (film in a camera is damaged by X-rays).

It is these properties that make them useful as a diagnostic tool.

ITQ 90 Give two properties of waves of the electromagnetic spectrum.

1.

2.

ITQ 91 In terms of energy waves, what is meant by:

a. Wavelength?

b. Frequency?

ITQ 92

X-rays have .... frequency and .... wavelength,

and are therefore .... energy waves.

ITQ 93 What are X-ray photons and where are they produced?

X-ray Machines

X-ray machines can be portable, mobile or fixed. All have an X-ray head and control panel. The head encloses an electrical transformer and X-ray tube. The electric current from the mains is transformed into a current of high voltage (measured in kilovolts) and low amperage (measured in milliamps). This new current passes through an X-ray tube resulting in the production of X-rays.

X-ray photons are produced in the X-ray tube by collision between fast-moving electrons and the atoms of another element, normally tungsten. Adjusting the settings on the machine can alter the intensity and quality of an X-ray beam. The X-rays produced in the head can only emerge from the tube via the window in the casing to form the **primary beam**. Any remaining X-rays are absorbed by the lead casing surrounding the X-ray tube.

The primary beam can be directed at the part of the patient needing investigation. X-rays penetrate skin and flesh whilst the denser structures of the body obstruct or absorb portions of the beam which causes a 'shadow' on the X-ray film. Radiography therefore shows changes in bone but not in soft tissue or cartilage.

Within the X-ray beam are some low-energy photons which are not powerful enough to pass through the patient, but which may be absorbed or scattered, hence representing a safety hazard (see Safety Issues, later this section). An aluminium filter placed across the window ensures the removal of these low-energy photons.

Also, during exposure, a further proportion of X-ray photons are not absorbed and do not pass through the patient, but are scattered. This scattering occurs when photons interact with tissue, lose energy and 'bounce' off in random directions. It increases when higher voltage is required to penetrate denser or thicker tissue. This is known as **scattered** or **secondary radiation** and is a potential hazard to the attendants, as well as blurring or fogging the X-ray film.

Scattered radiation can be reduced by:

1. **Collimation** or restriction of the primary beam by using a light beam diaphragm.
2. Use of the lowest necessary voltage.
3. A thin layer of sheet lead placed behind the X-ray film.
4. Use of a grid in front of the film. This allows X-rays through in one direction only.

The X-ray film, lead sheet and grid are usually contained within a cassette – a strong, durable, light-proof metal container designed to protect the film.

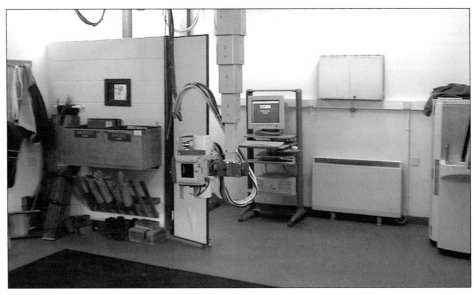

Figure 19 A fixed X-ray machine

ITQ 94 What is meant by the primary beam?

ITQ 95

a. What is it called when X-ray photons are not absorbed and 'bounce' off tissue in random directions?

b. What are the two main problems associated with this?
1.
2.

Formation and Interpretation of the X-ray Image (Radiograph)

The cassette is placed behind the area being X-rayed. The X-ray machine is positioned at a critical distance from the area. Several views are usually needed to provide an accurate investigation of the area. It is desirable to have the shortest exposure time possible to release the least amount of radiation and decrease the possibility of motion within the films (movement blur). Since any movement may void or blur the radiograph, the horse should be adequately restrained either physically or by sedation. (An additional reason for restraint is that a fractious horse may damage the equipment or injure handlers.)

The X-ray film is developed and can then be viewed on a screen. When developed, the X-ray is a picture in black, white and shades of grey. This is caused by the varying degrees of absorption of the beam by different tissues and hence differences in the amount of radiation reaching the X-ray film and causing blackening. For example, X-ray photons passing through bone will largely be absorbed and result in white areas, while X-ray photons passing outside the bone will blacken the developed film. Consequently, if X-rays are taken at the correct angle, fractures will be seen as black/grey areas in the bone. Cartilage is radiolucent, so will not show up on radiographs.

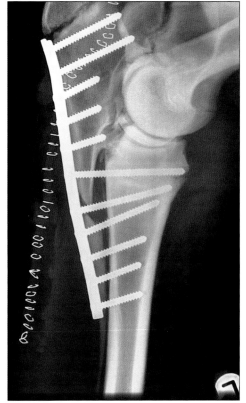

Although bone changes can appear dramatic, in many cases they are subtle and a trained eye is required to interpret the image.

In addition to diagnostic use, radiography is used following fracture surgery to monitor healing.

Figure 20 Radiograph showing internal fixation of a fractured elbow

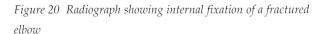

> **ITQ 96** A radiograph will show areas of black, white and shades of grey. Why is this?

Safety Issues

X-rays are invisible and painless, but their effects are both latent (i.e. may not manifest themselves until some time later) and cumulative. Safety must be taken very seriously when radiography is performed because radiation in various forms is potentially very hazardous and may even prove fatal.

THE EFFECTS OF RADIATION

The effects of radiation on living tissue are dependent on several factors:

1. The strength of the radiation.
2. The length of exposure.
3. How much of the tissue is exposed.

The tissues of the young are very susceptible to the effects of radiation and for this reason no person under the age of 16 or any expectant mother should be exposed to X-rays.

Whilst brief exposure to a low level of radiation is unlikely to cause damage, high levels of radiation, or repeated or prolonged exposure to low levels, causes the following types of changes:

Somatic – direct changes in body tissue after exposure. For example skin reddening and cracking, destruction of blood cells, baldness, cataract formation, damage to the reproductive organs and digestive upsets.

Carcinogenic – induction of cancerous tumours in tissue.

Genetic – mutations in chromosomes may occur, which may give rise to inherited abnormalities in offspring.

Because of the severity of the changes radiation can potentially induce, it is imperative that radiography is performed in an adequately protective environment.

PROTECTIVE MEASURES

1. **Dedicated room**. A specific room is identified for radiography to be performed in, and this should have sufficiently thick walls. A warning sign should be placed at the entrance to the room, consisting of a warning symbol (see Figure 21) and a sign saying 'controlled area'. It is also beneficial to have a red light outside the room to indicate that personnel should not enter when radiography is in progress. With portable machines, the controlled area is defined as the area within 2 m of the centre of the main beam. The vet is responsible for ensuring the safety of all personnel.

2. **Protective clothing**. This consists of aprons and gloves (or, alternatively, sleeves), usually made of plastic or rubber impregnated with lead (0.25–0.5 mm lead thickness). This will only protect against scatter and *not* against the primary

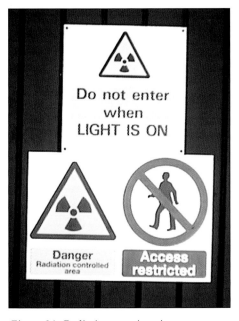

Figure 21 Radiation warning signs

beam. Aprons cover the trunk, especially the gonads, and should reach down to mid-thigh level at least. Single-sided aprons are cheaper and more comfortable but provide less protection. Gloves/sleeves are only necessary where manual restraint of the patient is required or if the cassette needs to be held.

Veterinary staff are required to wear radiation exposure badges, which measure radiation as the individual is exposed to it.

The minimum number of people should be present during exposure, and designated persons only (i.e. correctly trained personnel) are allowed to carry out the exposure.

ITQ 97

a. Why is prolonged or repeated exposure to radiation potentially dangerous to operators?

b. Which categories of person should not be exposed to X-rays?

c. Why is this?

ITQ 98 What precautions should be taken as protection against scattered radiation?

ULTRASONOGRAPHY

Soft tissues, such as tendons and ligaments, can be examined using the diagnostic ultrasound technique. High-frequency sound waves are transmitted from a **transducer**, which are then reflected off different tissues. The energy of the reflected waves is received by the **scanner** and changed electronically into a picture, which is displayed on the monitor.

The denser the tissue, the more resistant it is to sound waves. The sound waves bounce off the dense tissue structures causing an 'echo' (hence the use of ultrasound is termed **echography**). The denser the structures, the greyer the image seen on the screen. This is called **echogenicity**.

Sound waves will pass freely through blood or oedema (tissue fluid), showing up as a black area on the screen because they have not produced an echo.

For most scanning procedures the horse is normally placed in stocks and sedated. The area to be scanned is usually clipped and scrubbed to improve contact, and coupling gel is applied.

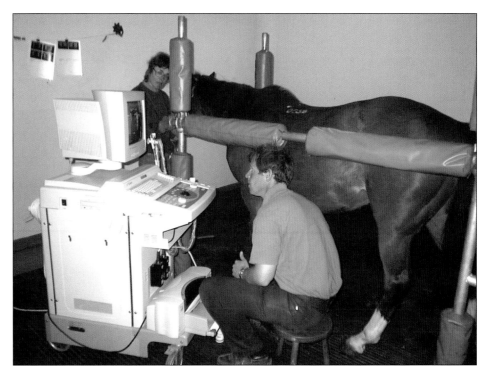

Figure 22 Ultrasound scanning

A common area for examination is the palmar (back) surface of the cannon bone where the tendons and ligaments can be seen. Imaging differentiates the various structures and allows evaluation of the tissues. The contralateral limb is often scanned as well so that a comparison can be made. Damaged structures are shown up as black areas as in Figure 23. This ultrasound picture shows a cross-sectional view – as if the lower leg was cut in half and you are looking down on the structures. By turning the hand-held transducer, the longitudinal view is shown. Both pictures would be used to assess the extent of the damage.

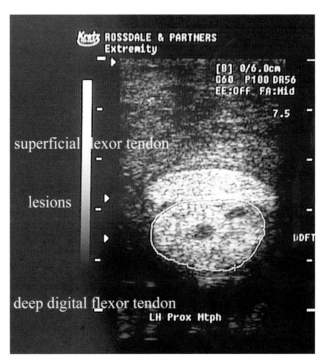

Figure 23 An ultrasound picture

Ultrasound scanning is also used to monitor the healing process. A horse may be sound, and the limb free from heat or swelling, but an injury may still not have healed fully. If a horse in this situation was brought back into work too early the injury could recur. As healing progresses the image will become increasing grey, i.e. its echogenicity increases. It is normal to scan damaged tendons every two to three months to monitor healing.

(In addition to scanning the lower leg, ultrasound is used for the detection of single or twin pregnancies, and for abnormalities of the reproductive tract, when the probe is inserted into the rectum. It is also a useful non-invasive technique in the diagnosis of colic, to ascertain the extent of any fluid-filled distensions of the gut.)

ITQ 99 Why is ultrasonography also referred to as echography?

NUCLEAR SCINTIGRAPHY

Gamma scintigraphy is used for the assessment of bone lesions, which do not always show up on X-ray. A radioactive substance (radioisotope), usually **technetium**, is injected intravenously, making the horse radioactive for a short time. The radioisotope is coupled to a bone-seeking agent called **MDP**. When injected, the technetium-MDP binds to actively metabolizing bone. At sites of increased bone turnover (such as a crack or fracture) more radiation is emitted, which results in **hot spots**.

These 'hot spots' can be detected by a gamma camera and are seen on a scintigraphy picture, which is sometimes called a 'bone scan'. The 'hot spots' show up as red areas on the bone scan.

The technique is different from X-raying. 'Hot spots' shown on the scintigraphy picture represent bone turnover at the time of examination; a radiograph is an image of what has happened in the past.

The technetium radioisotope has a half-life of 6 hours. (This is the time taken for half the radiation to disappear.) A short half-life is long enough to take a picture, but the radioisotope then decays rapidly.

By law, horses must be hospitalized during the period when they are radioactive, which should only occur at licensed premises. This is normally for a maximum of 36 hours post-injection. Minimum handling occurs and contaminated bedding should be left in the stable until it is safe to remove (urine and faeces will be radioactive for 36 hours).

As well as helping to diagnose a bone problem, nuclear scintigraphy is also a useful aid in monitoring the healing process. The main disadvantages of this technique are the cost of the equipment and the possible exposure risk to the handlers.

THERMOGRAPHY

Infrared thermography is a technique whereby measurements are made of the infrared emissions from an area and converted to a graphical representation (thermograph) on a screen. These thermographs are a quantitative representation of the area's surface temperature. Any increase in circulation and metabolism, e.g. in an area of inflammation, is shown as an increase in temperature, which, as in nuclear scintigraphy, is known as a 'hot spot'. This can be of some use in diagnosing lameness or injury, although this technique can prove unreliable.

ARTHROSCOPY

An area may need to be investigated surgically to determine the exact nature of the problem. An arthroscope is a narrow viewing tube that can be inserted into a joint through a small incision.

EXAMINATION PER RECTUM

This may prove useful in the diagnosis of diseases which may affect the pelvic and abdominal cavities, thus causing lameness.

ITQ 100 Name two diagnostic techniques that can be employed to diagnose problems associated with bone.

1.
2.

ITQ 101 Which diagnostic technique is only used in the diagnosis of problems associated with soft tissue damage?

CAUSES OF LAMENESS

We'll now look at some of the major causes of lameness in the horse.

SYNOVIAL AND BURSAL ENLARGEMENTS

The horse's limbs are susceptible to a range of soft swellings associated with synovial joints, bursae and/or tendon sheaths.

Synovial joints are joints encased in a capsular ligament forming a fibrous sac. The sac is lined by a synovial membrane that secretes synovial fluid. In response to stress, the synovial membrane may produce excessive synovial fluid, causing the joint sac to become distended, forming a soft, fluid-filled swelling, without heat or lameness. These swellings are classified as synovial enlargements or effusions.

Bursae are closed sacs lined by smooth cells (resembling the synovial membrane) which secrete synovial fluid. There are two types of bursae:

Congenital bursae – those which develop before birth, and are located in a constant position between structures where pressure is likely to occur, such as:

- Between a tendon or muscle and bony prominence (e.g. the navicular bursa).
- Between fascia and harder tissue.
- Between skin and underlying fascia joints.

Their functions are to allow free movement between the structures and to reduce strain, tearing and friction.

Acquired bursae – those which develop over bony prominences in response to trauma, such as capped elbow.

Tendon sheaths are long sacs lined by a synovial membrane which secretes synovial fluid to aid movement of the tendon: tendons are either fully or partially enclosed within a tendon sheath. If the synovial membrane becomes inflamed it will secrete excess synovial fluid and the sheath will become distended and swollen. The sheath may become permanently thickened and swollen once the inflammatory phase has passed.

Before we look at specific conditions associated with synovial and bursal enlargements, it should be appreciated that while some (especially those associated with infection and inflammation) can cause serious lameness, others do not cause lameness at all and are best left alone. Whilst it must be understood that a horse with the latter sort of enlargements has been subjected to a degree of 'wear and tear', he may be perfectly sound and fit for work. That said, if examining a horse prior to purchase with a view to competitive jumping, *any* swellings should be investigated carefully, as they *may* be indicative of arthritic changes occurring within the joint. However, the only competitive classes in which the horse may be marked down on the swellings alone are showing classes, where clean limbs are a prerequisite.

ITQ 102 What are the main functions of congenital bursae?

ITQ 103 Name two types of acquired bursae.

1.

2.

Bog Spavin

This is an enlargement of the tibiotarsal joint capsule; one or both hocks may be affected.

Dorsomedial aspect   Lateral aspect

Figure 24 Bog spavin

CAUSES

- Poor conformation (cow, sickle and/or straight hocks).
- Trauma (sprain).

(It should be noted that bone spavin and OCD (osteochondrosis dissecans) can also cause enlargement of the tibiotarsal joint but these conditions will also cause lameness, inflammation and/or radiographic changes.)

SIGNS

A soft swelling found on the front inner aspect of the hock and slightly higher up on the outside of the hock.

TREATMENT

No treatment is necessary, although topical applications such as Tensolvet (an anti-inflammatory that is readily absorbed through the skin), may help reduce the swelling. In certain cases the swelling subsides on its own.

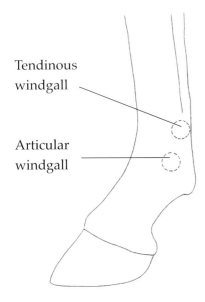

Tendinous windgall

Articular windgall

Windgalls

Windgalls normally form on one or both sides of the fetlock joint, being more common on the hind legs.

- An **articular windgall** is a distension of the fetlock joint capsule.
- A **tendinous windgall** refers to enlargement of the digital flexor tendon sheath.

Windgalls are cold, painless swellings not associated with lameness and no treatment is necessary.

Figure 25 Windgalls

ITQ 104 Complete the sentences.

a. An articular windgall is a distension of...

b. A tendinous windgall is an enlargement of...

Thoroughpin

This results from swelling of the tendon sheath enclosing the deep flexor tendon as it passes over the hock.

CAUSES

- Wear and tear.
- Strain.

SIGNS

- The swelling is seen on the inner and outer side of the hock and can often be pushed through the hock, which is why it is so named.
- The swelling is cold and is positioned higher than a bog spavin.

TREATMENT

Although treatment is not normally necessary, topical applications such as Tensolvet may reduce swelling. In some cases, the swelling may be resorbed naturally.

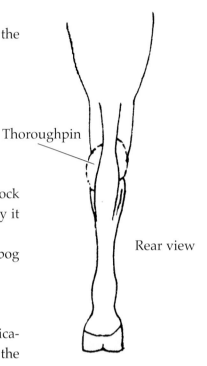

Thoroughpin

Rear view

Figure 26 Thoroughpin

Capped Knee, Elbow, Hock

A capped knee is sometimes called hygroma. Although unsightly, it rarely affects the horse's action. The 'capping' of these three joints has fundamentally similar causes (bangs or rubs) and treatments.

CAUSES (KNEE)

- Banging on the stable door.
- Hitting a fence.
- Inadequate bedding.

CAUSES (ELBOW/HOCK)

- Rubbing when the horse is lying down on thin bedding.
- Sometimes the elbow is capped when the horse lies down and the elbow rests on the shoe of a forefoot.

SIGNS

The front of the knee is enlarged and thickened; thickened swelling over the point of elbow or hock.

TREATMENT

1. Anti-inflammatory topical application may help reduce swelling.
2. Massage with an embrocation may help alleviate the effects but, once formed, there is very little to be done.
3. If the elbow becomes sore, a sausage boot can be fitted around the pastern, to help stop the heel of the shoe rubbing.
4. Make sure that the horse always has a good, thick bed.

PREVENTION

1. Remove any likely cause, e.g. pad the stable door with rubber matting.
2. Provide a good, deep bed.

Joint capsules and bursae are susceptible to injury and infection.

Synovitis

This condition results in inflammation of the synovial membrane lining a joint cavity. The membrane becomes thickened and secretes an excessive amount of synovial fluid into the joint. When the joint capsule is inflamed the condition is referred to as **capsulitis**.

CAUSES

- Injury – a sprain may occur as a result of the horse twisting suddenly.
- Infection.

SIGNS

- The joint is hot, painful and swollen, and may be kept flexed, with the toe resting on the ground.
- The degree of lameness will be determined by the extent of the inflammation.

TREATMENT

1. Rest the horse.
2. Consult the vet urgently.
3. The horse is likely to be admitted to an equine veterinary hospital for treatment.
4. If synovitis results from infection, the vet may flush the joint and administer antibiotics. It is important to reduce inflammation and flush out the infected joint because by-products of the inflammatory response and bacterial toxins are destructive to the articular cartilage. If untreated, degenerative joint disease (DJD) will ensue. (This condition is dealt with later on in this chapter.)
5. Cold treatments and bandaging may help alleviate the condition.
6. Consult a specialist regarding ultrasound, magnetic field or similar therapies.
7. The vet is likely to prescribe phenylbutazone to reduce inflammation and ease the pain.

Bursitis

This condition involves inflammation of a bursa.

CAUSES

- Infection – this may occur as a result of a puncture wound and is a dangerous condition.
- Trauma – a kick or blow sustained whilst working.

SIGNS

- Lameness.
- Visible swelling if the affected bursa is on a joint.
- If the affected bursa is within the foot, e.g. the navicular bursa, the lower limb will become swollen.

TREATMENT

1. Box rest.
2. Consult the vet, who will probably prescribe phenylbutazone to reduce inflammation and pain.
3. If the bursa is infected the condition is extremely serious – intensive antibiotic therapy will be needed and surgical flushing may be necessary.

DISORDERS OF BONE
Periostitis

The periosteum is the thin membrane that covers bone. As a result of a direct blow or damage to attached ligaments, the periosteum may become inflamed. This leads to haemorrhage beneath the periosteum, causing it to lift away from the bone. Bone-forming cells called osteoblasts respond by producing new bone. The main examples of periostitis in the horse are **splints** and **sore shins**.

CAUSES OF SPLINTS

Each splint bone is attached to the cannon bone by an interosseus ligament. As a result of friction and concussion, strain and tearing of this ligament occurs, which results in bleeding. The periosteum of the splint bone becomes inflamed and new bone is produced, forming a bony lump. Once formed, splints are not usually a problem unless a tendon or ligament rubs on the lump, or there is interference with a joint.

Splints are most often seen in young horses, whose bones are still developing, when their limbs are subjected to undue stress and concussion, e.g. caused by working on hard ground. Poor conformation, e.g. toe-in and bench knees, and incorrect trimming of the foot, resulting in poor hoof balance, can contribute to the development of splints, which can also be caused by a direct blow to the splint bone.

SIGNS

- Bony lump, most commonly seen on the medial aspect of the foreleg 6–7 cm ($2\frac{1}{2}$ in) below the knee.
- Heat, pain and swelling whilst forming.
- Varying degrees of lameness.

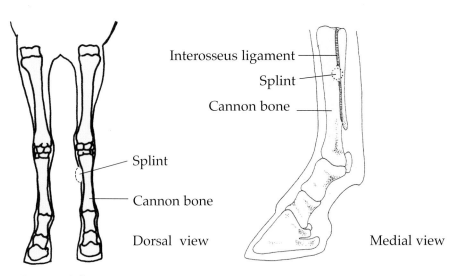

Figure 27 Splint

TREATMENT

1. Cold treatment to reduce inflammation.
2. Support bandaging to control inflammation.
3. Box rest to prevent aggravation.
4. Anti-inflammatories such as phenylbutazone may be prescribed.
5. Topical anti-inflammatory.
6. Surgery may be needed if the splint interferes with the suspensory ligaments or knee joint.
7. Extracorporeal shockwave therapy – shockwaves are high-energy sound waves transmitted to the affected area.

PREVENTION

- Do not work a young horse too hard, too soon, especially on hard ground.
- Always work horses in protective brushing boots.
- Keep the horse's feet correctly trimmed and shod to ensure good foot balance.

CAUSES OF SORE (BUCKED) SHINS

Here, there is inflammation of the periosteum at the front of the cannon bones of the forelegs. The condition is typically caused by concussion and is most usually observed in young Thoroughbreds in the early stages of race training (at 2 or 3 years of age) – it is not common in adult horses. As dirt tracks are used there, it is more common in the USA than in the UK. As the horse works, pressure and concussive forces are exerted on the dorsomedial cannon bone, and remodelling takes place. If the remodelling cannot keep pace with the repeated compression stresses, bone failure occurs. Microfracture and sub-periosteal haemorrhage result.

Direct trauma, perhaps from a kick, can also cause sore shins.

SIGNS

- Warm, painful swelling, usually on the front of both cannon bones of the forelegs. Severe cases with excessive swelling are known as 'bucked shins'.
- The stride may become shorter or the horse may appear obviously lame.

TREATMENT

1. A minimum of one month's rest is essential.
2. Cold treatments to reduce inflammation.
3. Specialist treatments such as shockwave therapy, laser or magnetic field therapy may be recommended by the vet/physiotherapist.
4. The vet is likely to prescribe non-steroidal anti-inflammatory drugs to reduce inflammation and pain.
5. The horse must be brought back into work in a controlled exercise programme to allow bone remodelling to keep up with the physical demands placed on the bone.

ITQ 105 What is periostitis?

ITQ 106

a. Give two examples of periostitis in the horse.

1.
2.

b. Give two causes of periostitis.

1.
2.

Ringbone

Ringbone occurs in four different forms:

1. **High articular (true) ringbone** – a degenerative disease of the pastern joint.
2. **Low articular ringbone** – a degenerative disease of the coffin joint.
3. **High non-articular (false) ringbone** – new bone formation on the distal (lower) end of the long pastern or on the proximal (upper) end of the short pastern. The joint is not involved.
4. **Low non-articular ringbone** – new bone formation on the distal end of the short pastern or the proximal aspect of the pedal bone, especially at the extensor process.

CAUSES

- Direct trauma to the bone.
- Tearing of the periosteal attachments of the collateral ligaments, extensor tendon or the joint capsule.

- Damage to the periosteum, e.g. puncture wound.
- Abnormal stress exerted by poor conformation, e.g. toe-in or toe-out.

SIGNS

Ringbone may be present in one or more fore- and/or hind limbs.

Articular ringbone

- The joint will feel hot.
- Reduced movement of the joint.
- Varying degrees of lameness, especially when the horse turns.
- Pain exhibited on flexion of the joint.

Non-articular ringbone

- Firm swelling in the pastern region.
- Initial lameness which usually passes as the inflammation subsides.
- High non-articular ringbone may be seen as a bony lump on the pastern.
- Low non-articular ringbone will need to be confirmed by X-ray.

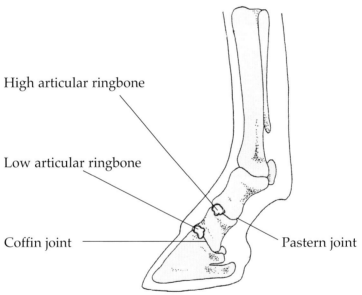

Figure 28 Articular ringbone

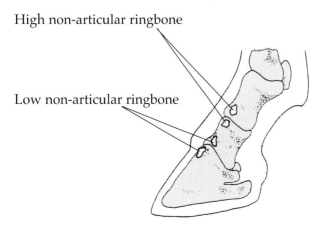

Figure 29 Non-articular ringbone

TREATMENT

1. Ringbone will have to be confirmed by nerve-blocking and radiography.
2. The vet may administer phenylbutazone in some cases.
3. Extracorporeal shockwave therapy.
4. The growth of new bone may lead to complete fusion of the joint, which may result in the horse coming sound, particularly if a hind leg is involved.

Sidebones

These bony lumps form as the lateral cartilages ossify (turn to bone).

CAUSES

- Concussion.
- Poor foot balance.
- Direct trauma to the lateral cartilages.
- Poor conformation, e.g. toe-in and toe-out.

SIGNS

- Lameness and shortening of the stride while the bone is forming.
- The lateral cartilages extend backwards from either side of the pedal bone. Normally they feel springy when the area above the coronet, towards the heel, is pressed. However, when sidebones are present, this area feels rigid.
- As the sidebone is developing the horse will exhibit pain when pressure is exerted on the affected area.

TREATMENT

1. Attention must be paid to correcting foot balance.
2. Box rest during the inflammatory stage.
3. In many cases no other treatment is necessary.

Once the sidebone has formed the inflammation subsides and the horse usually regains soundness.

Bone Spavin

This is an arthritis (degeneration) of the lower hock joints, with new bone formation. It is a 'wear and tear' condition, accentuated by poor conformation (sickle and cow hocks).

SIGNS

- Stiffness of the hind limb(s) when moving. This may wear off during exercise; however, stiffness worsens after hard work.
- Lameness will be accentuated after the hock has been flexion-tested.
- Lameness may be more noticeable if exercise is irregular.
- The horse may drag the toe of the affected limb(s), which leads to abnormal wearing of the shoe(s).
- The horse may be reluctant to flex the hock joint when his feet are being picked out, or for shoeing.

- The horse may start to refuse when jumping. Alternatively, he might want to stand off and jump flat, or get in close and jump off his forehand.
- Swelling may be seen on the front lower part of the inside of the hock.
- If one hock only is affected there may be muscle wastage on the affected side.
- Radiographic changes may show spurs of new bone, roughening of the bone contours and/or decreased bone density.

TREATMENT

1. Therapeutic shoeing (raised heel and rolled toe) may be recommended by the farrier.
2. Anti-inflammatory drugs, e.g. phenylbutazone may be prescribed by the vet.
3. Extracorporeal shockwave therapy.
4. Depending on the nature of the degeneration, surgery may be an option.
5. Despite numerous treatment processes, approximately half of affected horses remain lame and unusable. In some cases, however, treatment can prove highly effective.

Navicular Syndrome

This condition is progressively degenerative in nature and usually affects the navicular bones of both forefeet. The exact causes are not definitely known – the condition rarely appears suddenly but tends to be insidious in onset. Often, because the condition and therefore the lameness is bilateral (occurs in both forefeet), it may be well established before the owner is aware that there is a problem.

The condition occurs typically in horses between the ages of 7 and 12 years, is most common in Thoroughbred crosses and occurs more frequently in male horses. It is very rare in pure-bred Arabs or native ponies. Horses who have been subjected to high levels of work tend to be affected more frequently.

CAUSES

As stated, the exact mechanism of the condition is unknown. As opposed to there being one set cause, there are several factors which may predispose towards the onset of navicular syndrome.

- One theory is that it starts with a passive venous congestion within the foot (which may be caused by enforced rest). This congestion leads to increased blood pressure within the bone and thrombosis (clotting) within the arteries. This obstructs the flow of blood through the navicular bone – this condition, known as **ischaemia**, deprives the bone of essential nutrients and oxygen. This results in the death of small areas of the bone and ulceration, pitting and roughening of the cartilage.

    The deep digital flexor tendon passes over the cartilage on the back of the navicular bone, cushioned by the navicular bursa, before attaching to the lower aspect of the pedal bone. It applies pressure to the flexor surface of the navicular bone where the most significant lesions (pitting and roughening) occur. This causes trauma and pain to the deep digital flexor tendon.

- Another possibility is that the constant pressure exerted by the deep digital flexor tendon on the navicular bone compromises blood flow through the bone. This pressure is increased when shoeing is neglected and the pastern/foot axes becomes too sloping, with the toes long and the heels low and collapsed. It has also been suggested that the pressure causes bursitis within the navicular bursa and this inflammatory reaction leads to an alteration of the flexor surface of the bone.

- Hereditary defects such as conformational faults of the limbs, for example boxy feet, poor pastern/foot axes, excessively sloping pasterns and collapsed heels. These factors all add to the strain on the deep flexor tendons. Small feet and/or a large body can exacerbate the syndrome.

- The formation of sidebones results in a loss of elasticity in the foot and impaired circulation.

- Repeated compression and concussion from the frog below.

SIGNS

- Characteristically, the lameness first shows periodically and lasts for a short time only. Sometimes the lameness wears off with exercise. Lameness may show up more clearly after approximately 30 minutes rest following strenuous exercise.

- In the early stages the stride shortens gradually – because this happens bilaterally it may not be noticed immediately.

- The horse will tend to put the toe to the ground first before rapidly transferring his weight to the heel, resulting in a jarring appearance to the stride. The toe of the shoe will usually show signs of excessive wear. The shuffling gait often leads the owner to believe that the lameness is in the shoulder.

- As the condition progresses, the periods of lameness increase in duration and become more frequent. The horse may be prone to stumbling, although stumbling in isolation is not considered a sign of navicular syndrome.

- When observed in the stable, the horse may be seen trying to alleviate any pressure on the heels by standing with one toe pointing forwards. There may or may not be heat in the foot. The horse may shift his weight alternately from one foot to the other and dig the bedding in order to stand with his toes down and heels raised on a mound of bedding.

- The digital blood vessels may be enlarged as they pass over the sesamoids, but usually no increased pulsation is evident. By placing one's thumbs into the hollow of the heels and applying firm pressure, pain in the navicular area may be noted.

- Occasionally, the condition may affect one forefoot only – possibly as the result of bearing extra strain at a time when the other foreleg was suffering some form of injury, such as tendon strain. A severely affected foot may appear smaller than the other healthy forefoot, because of contraction of the heels.

- As the condition progresses the heels contract, causing the hoof to become upright and boxy.

DIAGNOSIS

- When tested for lameness, the horse suffering from navicular will normally demonstrate great discomfort upon continuous flexion of the fetlock and pastern joints. If trotted on immediately, exaggerated lameness, which gradually wears off, is usually seen.

- Navicular syndrome is diagnosed on the clinical signs and confirmed by selective nerve-blocking and X-ray. Palmar digital nerve-blocking will permit the horse to appear sound in the case of unilateral navicular syndrome. When both forefeet are affected, nerve-blocking of one foot will accentuate the lameness of the other.

  X-rays must be taken with the shoes off, the hooves must be very clean and the bottoms of the feet must be packed out to prevent shadows. Changes on the flexor surface are now thought to be the most significant.

- X-rays taken at approximately 4-monthly intervals will show pathological changes in the navicular bone and confirm the presence of the condition. The changes observed include the formation of extra nutrient foramina. (The various tissues of the body, including bone, contain many openings known as foramen, through which pass other structures such as blood vessels and nerves. In a normal working horse approximately five nutrient foramina, which should appear slightly conical in shape, may be seen along the flat lower edge of the navicular bone.) In the diseased bone, new blood vessels try to break through and supply the deprived area, increasing the overall number of openings and causing the existing foramina to become branch-shaped or rounded. On X-ray, changes in the shape of the foramina may be seen and any more than seven, or the appearance of foramina along the top or side edges, should be regarded as abnormal.

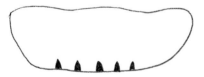

Normal nutrient foramina
of a healthy navicular bone

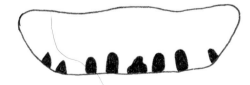

Abnormal foramina of a
diseased navicular bone

Figure 30 The navicular bone

ITQ 107 It is thought that venous congestion within the foot may be a contributory factor in navicular syndrome. Give two changes that occur as a result of venous congestion.

1.

2.

ITQ 108 Give two changes to the gait that occur when the horse suffers from navicular syndrome.

1.

2.

ITQ 109

a. What is ischaemia?

b. What effect does ischaemia have on the navicular bone?

ITQ 110 What causes the pain of navicular syndrome?

ITQ 111

a. What are foramina?

b. How do the foramina change when the horse suffers from navicular syndrome?

TREATMENT

The pathological condition cannot be treated – any damage to the bone and cartilage is usually irreparable. Treatment is aimed at relieving the pain and trying to extend the horse's useful life. No individual treatment can be relied on solely – the vet will make recommendations based on the individual case
Treatments include:

1. **Therapeutic shoeing**. When shoeing a horse suffering from navicular the aims are to relieve the pressure on the deep digital flexor tendons by encouraging straighter hoof/pastern axes, to promote improved circulation by increasing frog pressure and to ensure that each foot is properly balanced.

    The farrier may place the shoe well back under the toe, with the heels extending round to the back of the frog. Some may advocate the use of bar shoes, in particular the oval-shaped **egg-bar shoe** which is currently being used with some success. Pads or wedges may be used to raise the heels, thus easing pressure on the tendons and helping to reduce concussion. The heels are generally encouraged to grow downwards, which helps to straighten the hoof/pastern axes. It will be necessary to use rolled toes on the shoes to aid break-over.

2. **Vasodilator therapy**. Isoxsuprine hydrochloride is most effective in the very early stages of the disease, if the therapy begins immediately. Its main function is to widen blood vessels, thus allowing a free passage of blood. It is also thought to affect the viscosity of blood, acting as a thinning agent.

3. **Anticoagulant therapy**. One of the greatest breakthroughs in the treatment of navicular syndrome was the use of the anticoagulant drug, Warfarin. Warfarin reduces the viscosity of the blood, enabling it to flow through the affected vessels more easily, thus easing the state of thrombosis within the arteries. Because the treatment dose is close to the fatal dose, the dose rate has to be carefully calculated for each individual horse. The vet will take blood samples to ascertain the rate of blood-clotting.
Once dosing has started, blood samples are taken regularly to monitor the effect and to ensure that the safe level is not exceeded – an overdose could lead to haemorrhaging. The treatment often lasts for 9–12 months, in combination with corrective farriery and the introduction of regular exercise. Following this course of treatment, approximately 50 per cent of horses will stay sound. If lameness recurs, the treatment may start again.

4. **Anti-inflammatory drugs and analgesics**. Phenylbutazone (bute) has anti-inflammatory properties and is also analgesic. Of course, pain relief only masks the condition; it has no effect upon the degenerative process.
Another treatment is cortisone which, injected directly into the navicular bursa, may bring relief for between approximately 3 and 6 months.

5. **Extracorporeal shockwave therapy**. Shockwave therapy stimulates bone

formation and remodelling and many horses show improvement following treatment.

6. **Neurectomy**. Generally considered to be a last resort, neurectomy (or de-nerving) involves surgically removing part of the nerves supplying the heel region of the foot. This allows the horse to work for a few more months but eventually nerves either regenerate or form painful nerve-ending masses. Because of the way in which they grow back (in thread-like branches) the operation cannot normally be repeated.

A horse who has been 'denerved' must receive meticulous foot care as injuries such as puncture wounds may not be felt, and this can lead to infection and destruction of the foot structures without signs. FEI rules prohibit the use of neurectomized horses in competition.

7. **Desmotomy**. A relatively new treatment involves cutting the collateral (suspensory) ligaments of the navicular bone under general anaesthetic. The suspensory ligaments attach the upper border of the navicular bone to the long pastern. Desmotomy reduces the stress on the navicular bone and has improved the lameness in many cases.

ITQ 112 What are the three main aims when shoeing the horse with navicular syndrome?

1.
2.
3.

ITQ 113

a. Which drug may be used in the treatment of navicular syndrome to dilate the blood vessels?

b. What is the benefit of using an anticoagulant in the treatment of navicular syndrome?

c. Name the two surgical procedures that may be used in the treatment of navicular syndrome.
1.
2.

Pedal Ostitis

This term describes demineralization of the pedal bone and deposition of new bone as a result of chronic inflammation. Both forefeet are normally affected.

CAUSE

The commonest form of pedal ostitis is caused by concussion, which leads to chronic bruising and inflammation of the pedal bone and sole.

SIGNS

- Slight lameness, which improves with rest but recurs when work starts again.
- Shortening of the strides of the forelimbs on hard going – the horse will prefer working on soft ground rather than hard.
- X-rays will show distinct abnormalities in the bone's appearance – the outline of the bone becomes irregular and new bone is deposited on the front of the pedal bone.

TREATMENT

In serious cases, where new bone deposition is extensive and demineralization is great, the prognosis is poor and there is little to be done.

In less severe cases treatment may include the following:

1. Rest.
2. Shoeing to ensure straight pastern/hoof axes.
3. The farrier may recommend the use of a wide, flat shoe, the bearing surface of which is seated out to offer greater protection to the sole.
4. Exercise only on soft ground.

ITQ 114 What changes to the pedal bone can be seen on X-ray when the horse suffers from pedal ostitis?

Sesamoiditis

This term describes inflammation of the sesamoid bones, which may lead to the deposition of new bone, changes in bone density and/or an increase in the number of openings for blood vessels.

CAUSES

- Direct blow to the sesamoids.
- Concussion.
- Strain of the ligaments when the fetlock joint over-extends.

SIGNS

- Inflammation at the back of the fetlock joint.
- The horse reacts to firm pressure applied to the area.
- Varying degrees of lameness, which worsen on hard ground and at the start of exercise.
- If the fetlock joint is flexed for 1 or 2 minutes the horse will react, showing pain, and will trot up very lame.

- X-rays will show new bone deposition on the sesamoids or within the branches of the suspensory ligament.

TREATMENT

1. Cold hosing and support bandaging may reduce swelling in the acute stage.
2. Raised heels on shoes will reduce pressure on the fetlock joint.
3. The vet may prescribe anti-inflammatory drugs.
4. The horse will need a long period of rest – box rest for approximately 6 weeks.

Sesamoiditis has a tendency to recur.

LIGAMENT STRAINS
Curb

Curbs develop as a result of spraining the plantar tarsal ligament which runs down over the point of hock. They are found on the back of the hind leg, approximately 10 cm (4 in) below the point of hock. This swelling may become more fibrous with time. A **false curb** is a large head on the metatarsal (splint) bone, showing on the outside of the hock.

CAUSES

- Bad hock conformation, e.g. cow hocks and sickle hocks exert extra strain on the plantar ligaments.
- Strain caused by strenuous exercise.
- Stallions performing stud duties can be prone to curbs.

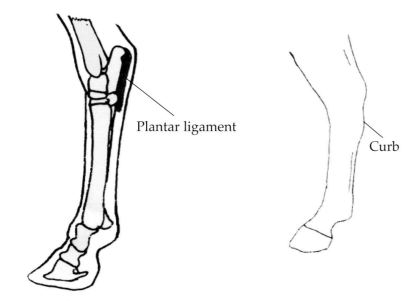

Plantar ligament

Curb

Figure 31 Curb

SIGNS

- The horse may or may not be lame.
- Heat.
- Swelling.
- The horse may stand with the heels slightly raised.

TREATMENT

- Rest.
- Cold therapy.
- Topical anti-inflammatories, e.g. Tensolvet. The vet may also prescribe phenylbutazone.

After treatment, the swelling tends to persist but does not cause any further problems

Suspensory Ligament Sprain
CAUSES

- Poor foot balance.
- Poor conformation, e.g. toe-in or toe-out.
- Fast work.

SIGNS

- Localized heat.
- Enlargement of the medial palmar vein on the inside of the leg.
- The ligament will feel softer and thicker than usual.
- When the limb is non-weightbearing, pressure applied to the ligament causes pain.
- Varying degrees of lameness, which may get worse after prolonged or hard work.
- The horse may be lamer on a circle than on a straight line.
- The horse may be lamer on a softer surface than on a hard surface.

TREATMENT

- Treatment is the same as for tendon injuries, i.e. rest, anti-inflammatory therapies and support.
- Extracorporeal shockwave therapy.

CONDITIONS AFFECTING JOINTS
Arthritis and Degenerative Joint Disease (DJD)

Arthritis is defined simply as inflammation of the joint which causes pain and stiffness. It is a non-specific term which may involve synovitis (inflammation of the joint lining) and/or be degenerative in nature. More specific terms are used to describe different types of the condition.

OSTEOARTHRITIS

When arthritis is degenerative in nature it is referred to as **osteoarthritis**, **arthrosis** or **degenerative joint disease** (**DJD**). DJD is the most common joint disease encountered in the horse, in particular the performance horse (for example, articular ringbone and bone spavin are forms of DJD). One or more of the following factors cause DJD to develop:

- Old age – a long period of wear and tear resulting from a normal workload.
- Cumulative effect of low-grade strains caused by poor conformation.

- Repeated loading of the joint as a result of a competitive discipline, e.g. jumping, polo.
- It can be secondary to other disorders or injury, e.g. joint infection, sprain, dislocation, fracture, osteochondrosis (see later this chapter).

In a healthy joint the bone ends are shaped to allow normal function and are covered in smooth cartilage – an organic matrix of collagen and **glycoproteins**. Collagen provides tensile strength; glycoproteins provide compressive stiffness. The whole joint is lubricated with synovial fluid; the main lubricant contained in both cartilage and synovial fluid is **hyaluronic acid**.

The onset of DJD causes a complex series of reactions to occur within the joint including the release of inflammatory mediators (enzymes and prostaglandins), reduction in articular blood flow and the over-production of synovial fluid which affects the hyaluronic acid balance. As joint lubrication is disrupted, the joint surface becomes progressively more ulcerated and decreased articular blood flow leads to damage of subchondral bone (bone below the cartilage).

In highly mobile joints (such as the fetlock, hock and knee) changes are first seen near the joint margins, and small bony projections (**osteophytes**) develop. As the disease progresses new bone may completely fill the joint space and this is termed **ankylosing arthritis**.

ANKYLOSING ARTHRITIS

In this form, destruction of the joint surfaces occurs, spurs of new bone develop around the joint and, because of the deposition of new bone, the joint capsule and ligaments become fused. This prevents movement (ankylosis). If ankylosis involves a low-motion joint (for example, bone spavin at a distal intertarsal joint), the lameness disappears once the ankylosis is complete. In a high-motion joint, however, crippling lameness may result, requiring veterinary opinion as to the benefits of carrying out treatment.

INFECTIVE (SEPTIC) ARTHRITIS

This is sometimes referred to as **joint-ill** or, if more than one joint is involved, **polyarthritis**. It is caused by bacteria gaining entry to the joints and must be treated as a medical emergency. In foals, the bacteria enter mainly via the navel and travel in the blood to the joint; in adult horses entry may be via a puncture wound.

Treatment of this form involves prompt and aggressive flushing of the joint with saline solution and extensive use of antibiotics to fight the infection, as the bacteria cause the joint surfaces to erode.

SIGNS OF ARTHRITIS

- Lameness, which may occur suddenly or gradually.
- Inflamed joint.
- Distension of the joint caused by increased production of synovial fluid.
- Difficulty in flexing the affected joint, giving a stiff appearance.
- Pain on flexion of the joint.
- Increased lameness after flexion-testing the affected joint.

- Infective arthritis is characterized by severe inflammation, pain and lameness.

DIAGNOSIS
- Clinical signs.
- Nerve-blocking.
- X-rays will show changes in bone, e.g. spurs and/or fragmentation at joint margins. X-rays will *not* show cartilage damage.
- Synovial fluid changes when DJD is present. Joint fluid can be drawn and examined.
- An arthroscope can be used to view the extent of the joint damage.

TREATMENT
The vet will determine the severity of the condition and decide on the most effective course of treatment. For example, if the arthritis has occurred as a result of infection, the horse will probably need to be admitted to an equine hospital for aggressive antibiotic treatment. Generally, treatment may involve the following:

1. Rest. Cease all hard work to allow the soft tissue inflammation to subside. If inflammation is acute the horse will need to be box-rested. On the vet's advice, walking in hand and passive joint manipulation may be carried out.

2. Phenylbutazone (bute), flunixin meglumine or meclofenamic acid may be prescribed to reduce inflammation and ease pain.

3. Extracorporeal shockwave therapy may be considered in some cases.

4. Two drugs used effectively to treat DJD are **Hylartil** and **Adequan**.
   Hylartil (hyaluronic acid) injected into the joint suppresses inflammation, improves synovial membrane function and replaces hyaluronic acid which has been broken down by the inflammatory response. It may prevent further cartilage damage but will not help repair existing damage. Three treatments given at 7-day intervals normally have a very good effect.

   Adequan (polysulphated glycosaminoglycan [PSGAG]), injected either intramuscularly or into the joint, inhibits destructive enzymes within the joint and promotes synthesis of hyaluronic acid. It is used in active synovitis and prevents cartilage degeneration. PSGAG can be injected intra-articularly once a week for up to five treatments. When administered intramuscularly a total of seven treatments can be given at 4-day intervals.

5. Intra-articular injections of cortisone reduces inflammation of the synovial membrane and controls the release of destructive enzymes. Research is ongoing as to the long-term effects of cortisone on cartilage.

6. A specialist may be consulted on the use of ultrasound, magnetic field therapy or similar.

7. Topical applications of Tensolvet may reduce soft tissue inflammation.

8. Cider vinegar mixed with cod liver oil may be added to the diet and does, in some cases, bring about improvement. There are several specifically prepared oils and additives that claim to aid joint mobility and reduce inflammation, and in certain cases they are helpful.

9. Corrective shoeing (raised heels and rolled toes) can ease strain on joints and improve break-over.

ITQ 115 What is the main lubricant within synovial fluid?

ITQ 116

a. What changes occur to the joint in DJD?

b. Give two alternative names for DJD.

ITQ 117 What happens to the joint in ankylosing arthritis?

ITQ 118 How is infective arthritis caused?

ITQ 119 Name two specific forms of DJD.

1.
2.

ITQ 120 What are the benefits of intra-articular cortisone injections?

ITQ 121 Name two drugs that are effective when injected intra-articularly.

1.
2.

ITQ 122

a. What are the main aims when shoeing the horse suffering from DJD?

b. How are these aims achieved?

Carpitis

In this condition the bones, ligaments or the joint capsule of the knee become inflamed.

CAUSES
- Direct injury, e.g. hitting a fence.
- Overwork of immature horses, e.g. racehorses.
- Faulty conformation of the knees.

SIGNS
- Lameness.
- Shortening of the stride.
- The horse may swing the leg outwards as the leg is drawn forward to avoid bending the knee.
- The horse will resent flexing the knee and lameness will be exaggerated after flexion-testing.
- The actual ability to flex the knee will be reduced.
- The affected joint capsule may be distended.

TREATMENT
1. Box rest with controlled walking in hand.
2. Anti-inflammatory drugs.
3. Cold therapies such as ice packs and hosing will help reduce swelling and pain.
4. Topical anti-inflammatory.
5. Other therapies such as laser, ultrasound and magnetic field therapy can aid recovery.
6. The joint should be flexed manually several times a day to prevent adhesions from forming.

Osteochondrosis

Osteochondrosis is a disturbance of conversion of cartilage to bone during bone formation, resulting in the persistence of cartilage in the area under the articular cartilage.

There may be separation of a fragment of articular cartilage and underlying bone. Such a fragment, referred to as a **joint mouse**, causes pain and varying degrees of lameness. Where such a fragment is present, the condition is referred to as **osteochondritis dissecans (OCD)**.

Young, rapidly growing horses are particularly susceptible. Youngsters being encouraged to grow quickly on a high nutritional plane, e.g. Throughbreds, are most at risk. Certain Warmbloods are also susceptible.

SIGNS

The condition is most commonly seen in one or both stifle or hock joints of young horses. It may also occur in the scapulohumeral (shoulder) joint.

- Osteochondrosis may show inflammation.
- The joint may be distended as a result of excessive synovial fluid production.
- Stiffness and/or lameness.
- Diagnosis will be confirmed by X-ray.

TREATMENT

1. If inflammation is present, anti-inflammatory therapy will be required. Because of the need for analgesia, phenylbutazone may be prescribed.
2. Where there is a fragment, surgery to remove it may be necessary to avoid development of DJD. In other cases, treatment is with rest and anti-inflammatories.
3. The long-term outcome depends upon whether or not DJD develops.

Intermittent Upward Fixation of the Patella

The stifle joint approximates to the human knee joint, and the patella approximates to the human kneecap. The stifle is the largest, weakest and most complex joint in the horse. Should the patella deviate from its normal position the joint may lock, forcing the limb to be held up in an abnormal way.

The normal locking mechanism, which the horse uses to rest whilst standing, involves locking the medial patellar ligament over the medial trochlear ridge of the femur. In upwards fixation, the patella becomes locked upwards and the releasing mechanism doesn't function properly.

CAUSES

- There is thought to be a hereditary basis for this condition.
- Conformation plays a significant role – a very steep angle between the femur and tibia will predispose the horse to this condition.
- Trauma.
- Young, unfit horses and ponies with poor muscle development are susceptible.

SIGNS

- The horse is not usually lame between episodes but the patella locks intermittently causing the hind leg to be held out with the hock and stifle locked.
- In mild cases the patella appears to 'catch' with each stride.
- In long-term cases the joint may become inflamed and the horse may become lame.
- DJD may develop.

TREATMENT

1. The stifle will normally unlock after a few strides. If it doesn't, pushing the horse backwards for a few steps usually has the desired effect.
2. Increase the horse's fitness and muscle tone with regular work.
3. Turn the horse out regularly.
4. If fittening the horse doesn't relieve the condition, the vet may cut the medial patellar ligament of the joint in a procedure called a **medial patella desmotomy**.

It is also possible, though rare, for the patella to become dislocated – this is sometimes referred to as a **slipped stifle**. Leading a horse carelessly through a partially opened stable door or gateway may cause the dislocation. The vet will be needed to correct the dislocation, reduce inflammation and promote muscle stimulation.

DISORDERS OF THE EXTERNAL STRUCTURES OF THE FOOT

Injuries to the foot are susceptible to invasion by tetanus bacteria. Therefore, whenever a horse suffers such an injury, it must be a priority to check that tetanus vaccinations are up to date. If they are not, consult the vet on this matter.

Sandcrack and Grasscracks

These are forms of damage to the hoof wall.

CAUSES

- Over-drying of the hoof in hot, dry weather.
- Shavings used as bedding material can dry out the hoof wall.
- General poor hoof condition caused by vitamin and mineral deficiency.
- Excessive rasping of the periople.
- Lack of hoof trimming.
- Poor hoof conformation, e.g. long toes and low heels.
- Chronic laminitis.
- Injury to the coronet, producing a weak, deformed hoof wall.

SIGNS

- A crack, which can vary from a hairline split to a deep shaft, running vertically up or down the wall. A crack originating at the coronary band is a **sandcrack**. Cracks originating at the ground surface are termed **grasscracks**.
- If very bad, a crack will pinch the underlying sensitive laminae, causing lameness.

TREATMENT

1. Consult the farrier, who will trim the hoof back properly.

2. The farrier may stop the crack from becoming worse by making a horizontal groove across the top or bottom (depending on origin). The horse may be shod with clips on either side of the crack to support the wall. The crack can be filled with the epoxy substance, Technovit.

3. Specially formulated additives are available, containing biotin and methionine, nutrients necessary for healthy hoof growth.

4. Prevent the hoof wall from drying out. There is a wide range of moisturising hoof creams available, although their efficacy is debatable.

5. If the crack is severe, it may be infected. The vet may be needed to administer antibiotics.

6. Animalintex poultices will help draw out any infection.

7. The crack may need to be widened to promote drainage.

Seedy Toe

In this condition, a cavity forms where the sensitive and insensitive laminae separate at the white line. The cavity fills with a 'cheesy', crumbly horn.

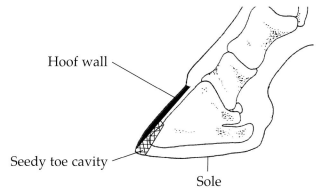

Hoof wall

Seedy toe cavity

Sole

Figure 32 Seedy toe

CAUSES

- Concussion of the toe area.
- Pressure from the toe clip following an infection after a sandcrack.
- Diseased laminae (the condition sometimes accompanies chronic laminitis).
- Alternate excessive dampness and dryness.

SIGNS

- The horn becomes brittle and crumbly, leaving a gap at the toe between the wall of the hoof and the laminae.
- The horse may be lame if the condition is severe.

TREATMENT

1. The cavity must be cleaned out and scrubbed, and packed with a substance such as cotton wool covered in Stockholm tar or a hard wax.

2. A wide-webbed shoe should be used to offer protection to the area.

Contracted Heels
CAUSES
- Boxy foot conformation.
- Poor shoeing.
- Drying out of the wall caused by removal of periople by excessive
- rasping.
- Lack of frog pressure, resulting in poor circulation.

SIGNS
- The heels of the foot become very narrow and contracted.

TREATMENT
A wide-webbed bar shoe (one with a large bearing surface) may be used to encourage the heels to spread and to promote frog pressure. If the cause has been poor shoeing in the past, consideration should be given as to whether a change of farrier is appropriate.

Thrush
Thrush is a condition arising from bad stable management – failure to pick out the feet daily combined with the horse standing in dirty / wet bedding, leading to a bacterial infection.

SIGNS
- Foul smell from the clefts of the frog.
- In severe cases, a black discharge will be present.
- If left unattended it may result in lameness as the frog becomes eroded and the underlying laminae damaged.

TREATMENT
1. Pick out and attend to the feet twice daily without fail.
2. Practise good stable management and ensure that the horse stands on clean, dry bedding.
3. Scrub the soles using an antibacterial solution such as Milton sterilizing solution.
4. Pack the clefts of the frog with Stockholm tar (which has antiseptic qualities) or, once the clefts are clean, spray liberally with an antibiotic spray.
5. If the infection has penetrated the underlying structures, the foot must be poulticed.

Bruised Sole
CAUSES
- Stepping on a sharp stone.
- Working on rough, uneven ground.
- Horses with flat soles and thin soles are very prone to bruised soles.
- Poor hoof balance may contribute.

SIGNS
- Varying degrees of lameness.
- Black/red/blue mark on the sole.
- Pain when pressure is applied by the hoof tester will cause the horse to flinch.

TREATMENT
1. Box rest on a non-heating diet.
2. A poultice, changed twice daily, will draw out the bruising. Once poulticing is finished, harden the foot off by spraying with gentian violet or antibiotic spray.
3. Antibiotics may be needed to fight infection.
4. The vet may prescribe phenylbutazone.
5. In a severe case, the farrier may cut out the bruise and fit a leather pad between the shoe and foot. Once the pad has been removed the farrier may suggest using a wide-webbed seated-out shoe.

PREVENTION
- Have the horse shod regularly.
- Never ride over very stony areas.
- Pick out feet twice daily to ensure that stones do not become wedged.

Corns

In the horse, corns are deep-seated bruising.

CAUSES
- Ill-fitting shoes, especially shoes that are too small.
- Shoes left on too long, resulting in pressure on the seat of corn (the area between the bar and the wall). Alternatively, a stone may have become wedged between the hoof and the shoe.
- Poor foot conformation – horses with flat feet and low heels are more likely to develop corns.

SIGNS
- Varying degrees of lameness.
- Bruising appears between the bar and the wall. In severe cases the sensitive laminae will also be bruised, which will cause great pain and lameness.
- The horse reacts to the application of pressure by the hoof testers.
- Infection may be present.

TREATMENT
1. Call either the vet or farrier to remove the shoe and relieve the pressure. They may pare away a small part of the bruised area.
2. If the corn is infected, poulticing will be necessary to draw out the pus. Healing must occur from the inside out to prevent infection being trapped within the hole.
3. The farrier may choose to use a leather pad between the shoe and the foot to offer full protection.

DISORDERS OF THE INTERNAL STRUCTURES OF THE FOOT
Nail Prick
CAUSE
The farrier nails too close to the white line and penetrates the sensitive laminae. This may happen if the horse moves suddenly during nailing on.

SIGNS
- The horse will flinch as the nail penetrates the sensitive laminae during shoeing.
- The farrier usually realizes that the horse has been 'pricked'.
- As the nail is pulled out there may be slight bleeding.
- If the nail is not withdrawn straight away the horse will be acutely lame immediately.

TREATMENT
1. Flush the hole with Pevidine solution.
2. Apply an Animalintex poultice.
3. Box-rest for a few days to minimize the risk of contamination.
4. If the horse becomes lame and/or the hoof wall feels warmer than normal, consult the vet as infection may be developing within the foot.

Nail Bind
CAUSE
A nail is driven too close to the sensitive laminae, causing great pressure.

SIGNS
- The horse will become lame hours, or even days, after shoeing.
- Possibly heat in the affected foot.
- The horse will react when the wall is tapped lightly in the region with a hammer.

TREATMENT
1. Either the vet or farrier should remove the nail.
2. Poultice the foot to help draw out any infection.
3. Rest the horse, as the area may be bruised.

Quittor
CAUSES
Injury or infection of the lateral cartilages.

SIGNS
- An abscess forms within the lateral cartilages and bursts above the coronary band.
- While the abscess is forming there will be heat and pain in the foot.
- The horse will be lame.

TREATMENT

1. Call the vet to draw out the infection and give an antibiotic injection.
2. As with a puncture wound, it is important that this wound heals from the inside out.

Laminitis

Laminitis is a complicated disease which can affect both horses and ponies, but more commonly affects the latter. Research continues in an effort to determine why some animals are more prone to the condition than others, and what exactly causes it. Studies by R.A. Eustace and P.J. Cripps (1999) recommend that the term laminitis should be further broken down to describe the condition more accurately. Based on the vet's clinical assessment, individual cases should be classified as laminitis, acute founder and sinker or chronic founder. These terms are described later. Prognosis is affected according to the category.

Laminitis occurs as a result of several physiological changes which take place throughout the body, all culminating in a displaced blood flow through the sensitive laminae of the hoof wall. Laminitis may affect any combination of fore or hind feet but, usually, both forefeet are involved.

There are three distinct phases of the disease:

1. **The developmental phase**. During this phase the horse is exposed to the factors that cause laminitis.

2. **The acute phase**. This phase starts as soon as the first sign of lameness is exhibited and lasts a variable amount of time.

3. **The chronic phase**. This starts as soon as there is rotation of the pedal bone or if the lameness has lasted more than 48 hours. The chronic phase can last for weeks, months or years.

The physiological changes that occur as the disease develops, and the rationale which Eustace and Cripps apply to classify individual cases, are outlined below.

THE PHYSIOLOGICAL EFFECTS OF LAMINITIS

With the onset of the condition the blood pressure rises, causing circulatory changes in the feet. This is not yet fully understood as, although the increase in blood pressure causes *increased* blood flow to the feet, the blood flow through the sensitive laminae is *decreased*. It is thought that blood is 'shunted' from arterioles to venules without passing through the capillary bed of the laminae.

There is a strong, bounding pulse in the digital arteries, level with the fetlock, partially the result of pain and the effect of the arterial blood reaching the obstructed vessels within the foot. (At this stage, by definition, the horse has **laminitis**.)

The capillary network within the sensitive laminae becomes congested with blood, the pooling of which results in the inefficient exchange of gases, leading to oxygen starvation in the tissue cells of the sensitive laminae. (The condition may be further complicated by **sporadic intravascular coagulation** – the pooling blood may clot in places, which further impedes the blood flow.) This deprivation of oxygen causes damage to the tissue, the severity of which depends on the length of time for which blood flow is disrupted. The inter-laminar bond supports the pedal bone – reduced blood flow damages this bond, leading to separation. When enough inter-laminar bonds are damaged the pedal bone drops within the hoof. The horse is then described as having **foundered**.

The weight of the horse bearing down on the pedal bone causes further separation. This, combined with the upward pull of the deep digital flexor tendon, causes the pedal bone to sink and/or rotate further. The blood vessels between the pedal bone and the sole become compressed, which may lead to the death of the tissue in the area (necrosis).

If not corrected, there is total destruction of the inter-laminar bonds and the pedal bone becomes totally loose within the hoof – the horse is then described as a **sinker**. The pedal bone may penetrate the sole in front of the point of frog. If this occurs, the prognosis is extremely poor and euthanasia should be considered. Any damage to the tissue of the sole may then lead to secondary infection of the sensitive laminae ('seedy toe'). The rotation of the pedal bone may lead to a convex appearance of the sole and severe lameness.

ITQ 123 List three circulatory changes that occur within the foot when the horse suffers from laminitis:

1.

2.

3.

ITQ 124 What causes rotation/dropping of the pedal bone?

CAUSES

As mentioned above, the exact causes are not known. However, laminitis may be divided into two categories:

- **Traumatic/mechanical laminitis** in which the physiological changes are not the primary cause. Concussion, e.g. jumping on hard ground, may cause bruising and damage to the tissue of the sensitive laminae, and improper foot trimming and shoeing resulting in pressure on the sole can lead to laminitis.

- **Systemic laminitis**, which is caused through a culmination of physiological changes in the body.

There are many different factors which, in any combination, may cause a reduction in blood flow through the vessels of the sensitive laminae, and trigger off systemic laminitis. These factors include:

1. **The production of endotoxins**, arising from circumstances such as:

- **Retained placenta**. Toxins are produced within the body as a result of a bacterial infection. For example, after foaling there may be retention of the placenta leading to infection of the uterus (endometritis).

- **Strangulating obstruction** (see Colic in Chapter 5). Endotoxins are released from compromised gut in a strangulating lesion.

- **Carbohydrate overload** from corn or spring grass (see Figure 33 next page). This alters the balance of bacteria within the caecum, resulting in the production of lactic acid. The change in pH kills some of the gram-negative bacteria with the resultant release of endotoxins. These are absorbed into the bloodstream, causing laminitis.

- **Liver disease**. If, for some reason, the liver is damaged and not functioning properly, endotoxins may build up in the circulation, causing laminitis. A blood test would show raised liver enzymes.

2. **Obesity**. Laminitis commonly occurs in obese horses and ponies.

3. **High doses of steroids** (cortisone) increase the response of the digital blood vessels to circulating levels of adrenalin. This may result in 'shunting' and reduced blood flow to the feet. Corticosteroids are used to treat a range of conditions, e.g. joint lameness and sweet itch, and can trigger an attack of laminitis. *Corticosteroids should never be used to treat laminitis.*

4. **Viral respiratory disease** that causes a great increase in body temperature can render the horse susceptible to laminitis. The first signs of laminitis may be seen some 2–3 weeks after the viral infection.

5. **Changes in the levels of hormones** produced by the endocrine glands. Marked changes in the levels of hormones including cortisol, testosterone, aldosterone, oestrogen, progesterone, renin and thyroxin could render the horse more susceptible to laminitis.

6. **Cushing's disease**, which is common in older horses, is caused by a benign tumour on the pituitary gland in the brain. One of the side effects of Cushing's disease is a 'high risk' of laminitis. The primary problem in this instance is a non-feed related laminitis, although these animals often respond well to a 'laminitic diet'.

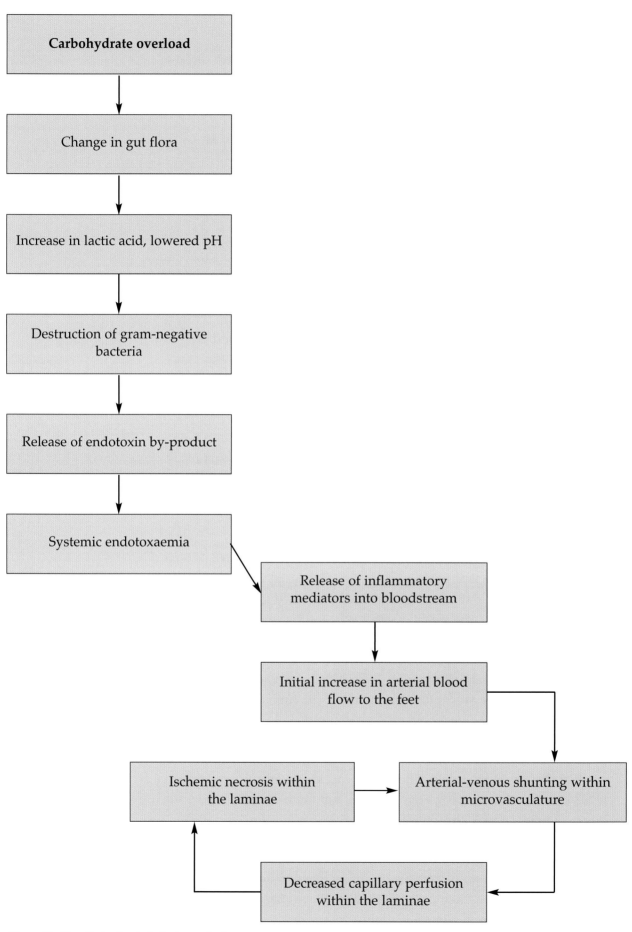

Figure 33 The effects of carbohydrate overload

7. **Stress**. Stress such as worming, overworking an unfit horse, prolonged transit and vaccination can trigger an attack.

8. **An imbalance of calcium to phosphorus and of sodium to potassium**. These imbalances are thought to affect the passage of electrochemical nerve impulses, which could cause paralysis of the muscles of the arterial walls – this would exacerbate the problem of increased blood pressure. Moreover, the balance of minerals in the body affects the metabolism, therefore a general mineral deficiency may predispose to laminitis.

> ITQ 125 List three causes of endotoxin production.
>
> 1.
> 2.
> 3.

SIGNS

Eustace and Cripps classify lameness associated with the various stages of laminitis in six stages:

Grade 0 No lameness at walk or trot on a straight line on a hard surface.

Grade 1 No lameness at walk; horse moves freely. Some lameness in trot and turns carefully.
Additionally:
- The horse may shift his weight from foot to foot to relieve the discomfort.
- Often, but not always, the feet feel warm, particularly around the area of the coronet.
- The horse is not lame but, at trot, has a short, choppy gait.

Grade 2 The horse moves stiffly at walk, moving with his weight back on his heels, and is unwilling to trot: turns with great difficulty.
Additionally:
- The horse will react when the hoof testers are applied just in front of the frog.
- At this stage many horses develop a characteristic 'sawhorse' stance – the weight is borne on the heels, with the hind feet well under the body and the forelegs extending forward.

Grade 3 The horse is reluctant to move, finding turning particularly difficult, and will resist attempts to have a foot lifted. The horse may be virtually non-weightbearing on one limb.

Grade 4 The horse will refuse to move without coercion and it is impossible to lift a limb.
Additionally:

- The horse may sweat and his breathing quicken.
- The horse may lie down and be reluctant to stand.
- There is a bounding digital pulse.
- The hoof walls may feel hot, particularly around the coronet.
- There may be a rise in temperature, which might go as high as 41 °C (106 °F). The pulse rate may increase to between 50 and 120 beats per minute because the horse is in extreme pain.

Grade 5 The horse spends most of his time recumbent and cannot stand for more than a few minutes.

TREATMENT

Because of the serious nature of this disease, the vet must be called for all but the mildest cases of laminitis. 'Mild' may be interpreted as the signs being spotted and treated very quickly (same day) followed by rapid improvement (next day) and no recurrence.

Treatment can be divided into three categories.

1. Removal of the primary cause

- Take the horse off grass and stable him on deep, non-edible bedding. Peat or shavings are ideal as these pack into the soles of the feet, providing support.

- The horse should receive only hay of good quality but low feed value, and water. Obese animals should have their food intake reduced gradually to avoid liver damage and hyperlipaemia. (The school of thought at one time was to feed bran mashes. This is now known to interfere further with the calcium:phosphorous ratio. Bran contains a high level of phosphorus and bran fibre inhibits the horse's ability to absorb and utilize calcium. Whenever bran, or indeed any grain, is fed, limestone flour or alfalfa should be added to boost calcium levels.)

- If the horse has eaten a large quantity of feed, perhaps as a result of escaping and gorging in the feed room, the vet may administer a solution of mineral oil (e.g. liquid paraffin) and electrolytes via a stomach tube. This acts as a bulk laxative, helps to flush out the digestive tract and prevents the absorption of endotoxins.

- Probiotics should be added to the feed to help re-establish the normal functioning of the gut flora.

- A mineral supplement containing biotin, methionine and zinc will help re-establish the depleted keratin sulphate of the laminae. A mineral lick should be available at all times.

- In the event of any infection, the vet will prescribe and administer the necessary antibiotics. If an infection is suspected, particularly in connection with a broodmare, the vet must be called immediately. (If the placenta has not been expelled within 10 hours, call the vet, who will administer oxytocin to stimulate uterine contractions).

2. **Correction of circulation and analgesia**
- The high blood pressure is partially a result of the great pain so, for the comfort of the horse, analgesia must be a priority. The vet will prescribe an analgesic such as **phenylbutazone**. Although research carried out has shown that this can affect the metabolism of sodium and potassium, it is still the number one choice. (However, it must only be administered to ponies under veterinary prescription. It is known to cause liver damage and has other side-effects in certain breeds of pony.)

- In endotoxaemic cases, a non-steroidal anti-inflammatory drug such as **flunixin meglumine** may be given intravenously, followed by oral administration. Flunixin is effective against bacterial toxins. (As mentioned earlier, corticosteroid anti-inflammatories are contra-indicated as they can actually *cause* laminitis and may make the situation worse.)

- The vet is likely to administer drugs which dilate blood vessels (**vasodilators**), thereby reducing blood pressure and easing congestion within the feet. Such drugs include acetyl-promazine (ACP) and phenoxybenzamine. ACP will also help calm the horse (in higher doses it acts as a sedative).

- **Anticoagulant therapy** e.g. aspirin and heparin has also been used. Careful monitoring of clotting ability is essential.

- Hosing or tubbing with warm water will help to relax and dilate the capillaries within the foot, so easing congestion. However, another traditional treatment, cold hosing, is now known to generally aggravate the condition. The application of cold water causes further vasoconstriction, impeding circulation. Nonetheless, in the very acute stage, cold hosing may assist insofar as it reduces the metabolic rate of the cells and thus reduces the tissues' demand for oxygen.

- Box rest will encourage the damaged laminitic tissue to repair and prevent further rotation. Walking exercise is now known to be of no benefit to the laminitic animal. The bed should be very deep to encourage the horse to lie down and keep the weight off his feet.

ITQ 126 Which non-steroidal anti-inflammatory drug is effective against bacterial toxins?

ITQ 127 What is the purpose of administering acetyl-promazine in the treatment of laminitis?

ITQ 128 Which type of drugs may be administered to aid the circulation of blood through the foot?

3. Prevention of pedal bone rotation/dropping

If the laminitis is at all prolonged (signs persist for 48 hours or longer), it will be necessary to have the feet X-rayed to determine whether the pedal bone has rotated and, if so, by how much. Only then can the vet and farrier plan a suitable programme of foot care. X-rays are taken at the start of treatment and then regularly to assess progress.

Prior to radiography the vet may tape a frog support pad over the frog to offer temporary support.

Metal markers are taped to the front of the hoof wall and 1 cm (0.4 in) behind the point of frog when the X-rays are taken to show the degree of rotation/dropping.

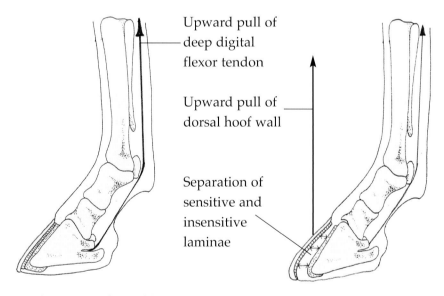

Upward pull of deep digital flexor tendon

Upward pull of dorsal hoof wall

Separation of sensitive and insensitive laminae

Normal position of pedal bone   Rotated pedal bone

Figure 34 Position of the pedal bone – normal and rotated

SUPPORTIVE FARRIERY

Once the stage of acute laminitis has passed, farriery can be carried out. The objectives of foot care in the chronic case are to:

• Maintain frog support.
• Reduce the tearing forces of the deep digital flexor tendon.

- Protect the integrity of the laminae.
- Provide drainage if infection is present.
- Remove necrotic tissue and debris.

The main aim of shoeing is to provide a therapeutic level of frog pressure. This is likely to involve:

- Trimming back the toe to help realign the contours of the hoof with the pedal bone. Shortening the toe also decreases the tension on the deep digital flexor tendon, which reduces its tearing forces.

- Lowering the heels gradually. If performed too quickly this can increase the tearing forces of the deep digital flexor tendon.

- The use of **heart-bar shoes**. Heart-bar shoes offer support to the pedal bone and take the pressure away from the toe, which allows the reattachment process to proceed unhindered. The heart-bar shoe must be fitted accurately. There must be a small gap between the ground surface of the frog and the 'V' section of the shoe to allow frog movement.

If the foot is too painful for normal shoeing, glue-on shoes can be used. An elevated heel shoe may be used to reduce the pull of the deep digital flexor tendon.

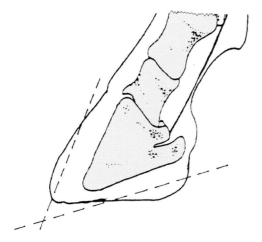

Figure 35 Corrective trimming to realign the pedal bone

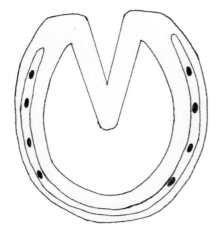

Figure 36 Heart-bar shoe

DORSAL WALL RESECTION

This procedure is carried out by the farrier under veterinary supervision.

Biomechanically, the dorsal hoof wall acts as a lever, increasing the tearing forces between it and the pedal bone. A dorsal wall resection involves removing the front of the hoof wall between the quarters to within approximately 1.5 cm (0.6 in) of the coronary band, down to the sensitive laminae. The objectives of this procedure are to:

- Lessen the biomechanical leverage effect of the hoof wall.
- Allow inflammatory exudate to escape, thus relieving pressure and pain.
- Ease the pressure from blood vessels supplying the coronary band.
- Encourage realignment of the pedal bone and hoof wall as the new wall grows parallel to the front of the pedal bone.

The sectioned area of the hoof will need to be kept scrupulously clean and covered with antiseptic bandages. Systemic antibiotics will be needed to counter infection.

This technique can be modified – the toe can be rasped to expose the sensitive laminae at the foot's most distal aspect. The portion of hoof near the coronary band is thinned. This too reduces the biomechanical forces acting on the hoof whilst maintaining structural integrity and reducing the risk of infection.

SURGICAL PROCEDURES

In chronic, severely rotated cases, the deep digital flexor tendon shortens, preventing realignment of the pedal bone. Some improvement may be achieved through cutting the deep digital flexor tendon (**tenotomy**) or its accessory ligament (**desmotomy**).

These procedures are only performed as a last resort – the horse will never be sound enough to resume work.

ITQ 129 List four objectives of foot care in a case of chronic laminitis.

1.
2.
3.
4.

ITQ 130 When trimming the laminitic horse's foot the farrier is likely to shorten the toe. What are the effects of this?

> ITQ 131 What is the main aim of shoeing the laminitic horse?

PROGNOSIS

Mild cases of laminitis tend to recover well if treated promptly. If an acute case of laminitis is not quickly resolved the prognosis is guarded. Once the horse has suffered one attack he will always be susceptible – the owner must be vigilant in the long-term management of such a horse.

Where pedal bone rotation occurs the foot care regime is of great importance. In many cases of severe rotation euthanasia is the only humane course of action to take.

PREVENTION

(These steps are sensible precautions, not guarantees of avoidance.)

- Restrict access to lush grass. Use electric fencing and/or stable the horse for several hours a day. Muzzling the horse allows him to drink but not eat. Grazing muzzles allow the horse to pull at grass but restrict the amount that can be eaten.
- Never over-feed carbohydrate-rich foods.
- Feed a balanced diet.
- Feed according to workload.
- Always keep the feed room door locked to prevent an escapee horse from gorging himself.
- Call the vet promptly to treat retained placenta and cases of colic.
- Avoid prolonged trotting on the roads.

CHAPTER SUMMARY

The subject of lameness in the horse is vast. This chapter has dealt with some of the causes of lameness – it has not attempted to cover the entire range of conditions. It is important that you are able to recognize the norm in terms of the horse's limbs and movement. This enables you to notice subtle changes promptly – in many conditions, the earlier the problem is caught, the greater the chance of full recovery.

Identifying lameness and its causes is an important aspect of horse management. The advice of the vet should be sought when the reason for the lameness is not obvious. The vet must always be called immediately if the horse is non-weightbearing on a limb, has sustained a puncture wound on a joint or to the sole or appears to be suffering from laminitis. These are emergency situations that can lead to permanent unsoundness.

CHAPTER 7

MANAGEMENT OF THE SICK OR INJURED HORSE

The aims and objectives of this chapter are to explain:

- The precautions that should be taken to control the spread of disease.
- How to care for the sick horse.
- Methods of administering medication.
- The basic principles of a rehabilitation programme.

CONTROLLING DISEASE
QUARANTINE AND ISOLATION

These terms refer to the separation and segregation of infected or potentially infective horses from those presumed to be free of infection. The term quarantine (originally a period of 40 days) is used more generally nowadays and, for our purposes, in relation to horses who are to be kept separated before travelling abroad and/or upon arrival at a new yard. In terms of import and export, quarantine regulations vary between countries. Yards receiving new horses, especially horses who have come from the sales or whose health status is unknown, should quarantine all new horses for approximately ten days before allowing them to mix, in case they are incubating an infectious disease.

Viral infections such as rhinopneumonitis and influenza, and bacterial infections such as strangles, can spread through a group of horses causing an epidemic. Horses who are known to have, or suspected of having, an infectious disease should be quarantined, as should horses who have had diarrhoea within the previous 24 hours or enlargement of the lymph nodes around the head.

All animals new to the yard should be inspected for respiratory disease and ringworm. A worm egg count can be carried out to determine the presence and type of worm infestation.

The Isolation Box/Yard

Such facilities allow for newly arrived horses to be housed away from the main stabling area for an interim period, and horses who contract any contagious or infectious disease can be stabled away from others to reduce the spread of the infection.

Every commercial yard should have at least one stable specially set aside for isolation/quarantine purposes. An isolation box is essential on yards requiring a Riding School Licence. Large establishments will have a smaller isolation yard equipped to deal with several horses. The yard should be clearly signed as an isolation facility with access restricted to authorized persons only.

The isolation facility should be sited as far away from the main stables as possible, ideally no closer than 80 m (90 yards) to the other stables. It should face away from the main stables, with the prevailing wind blowing from the stables towards the isolation facility. There should also be road access to the isolation facility so that horses can be unloaded or loaded close to the isolation area and so that the vet's car and equipment can be left close to the stable.

Each isolation box should also contain an area for all the equipment the horse and stable needs. This has to be large enough to contain feed, grooming kit, tack and mucking out equipment.

Isolation boxes should be constructed so that they can be easily disinfected after use. They should be made of brick rather than wood, as harmful organisms remain in wood for a longer time. Ideally, the brickwork should be rendered so that it can be kept as clean as possible. If possible there should be a water supply close to the box, so that cleaning the box after use can be carried out as easily as possible. There should be as little stable furniture as possible in the box (only a water bowl and tie ring), to prevent the build-up of harmful organisms.

There should also be a separate muck heap which may be burnt to destroy the soiled bedding.

Isolation Procedure

Once he is in isolation, the bedding in the horse's original stable must be burnt and the stable thoroughly disinfected. Each horse in isolation must have his own equipment such as mucking out tools, grooming kit, buckets and rugs. These must never be used on any other horses. All items should be labelled to avoid confusion. A good way of doing this is to put a small dab of brightly coloured paint or electrical (bandage) tape on everything. All grooming kit, rugs, numnahs and other items of clothing must be washed regularly in hot water and an appropriate disinfectant. **Virkon,** a broad-spectrum disinfectant effective against viral, bacterial and fungal organisms, is recommended by vets.

- In serious cases movement of horses on and off the premises must stop.

- If more than one horse is infected they must be isolated as a small group.

- Any animals who have been in contact with the infected horses are referred to as 'in-contacts' and should be isolated as a small group (away from the infected group).

The Handler

Ideally, one person should have the sole responsibility of caring for the sick horse. This lessens the chances of spreading the disease around the yard. If this is not possible, whoever is going to look after the sick horse must leave him until last.

A pair of overalls should be worn and the handler's head should be covered. The handler's boots must be dipped in a disinfectant boot dip before and after handling. Disposable boot covers and head covers should be provided.

Latex gloves should be worn and the handler's hands and arms must be scrubbed in hot, soapy water after handling. A waste disposal bin should be placed outside the stable for the disposal of disposable protective clothing.

Yard Hygiene

Large numbers of horses inevitably result in a large population of bacteria on the premises. These need not be detrimental to healthy horses but may present a challenge to a newborn foal or unhealthy adult horse. Hygiene plays a large part in the prevention and control of disease.

- Ideally, horses should be kept in small groups to minimize the bacterial build-up.

- Barren and maiden mares should be kept separate from pregnant mares and mares with foals at foot. Yearlings should not be kept with adult horses.

- Foaling boxes must be kept scrupulously clean – the walls and floor should be steam-cleaned and disinfected before the first mare uses the box and then again after she and each subsequent mare moves out.

> ITQ 132 What is meant by 'in-contacts' and how should they be treated?

ASPECTS OF MANAGEMENT
THE STABLE ENVIRONMENT

Generally when a horse is sick or injured, he will spend most of the time stabled to allow you to monitor his condition and maintain a high level of care. The stable must be scrupulously clean, with a good bed. The bedding must be clean, dry and dust-free. If the horse is well enough, lead him into a spare box (subject to same conditions as the isolation box) while you muck out. Pay great attention to hygiene in the stable, using a disinfectant to wash down the floor at least once a week. Remove cobwebs, as they attract dust.

When disinfecting a stable known to have housed a horse with an infectious condition the area immediately outside the stable door should be thoroughly soaked with disinfectant so that the wheelbarrow passes over the disinfectant. Remove all movable equipment such as feed bowls and water buckets. Remove bedding, making sure it cannot blow out of the wheelbarrow. Jet-wash the stable and allow it to dry before disinfecting the walls and floor. If disinfectant is applied to wet surfaces the water can form a barrier, preventing the disinfectant from acting on the surface behind.

Feed and water bowls should be washed with a Virkon solution, rinsed and allowed to dry before being put back into the stable.

Non-edible, low-dust bedding such as paper or shavings should be used to prevent the horse eating the bedding, which could lead to an impacted colic. If using shavings, bank up the sides of the bed well to exclude draughts and prevent the horse from becoming cast when he lies down. If the horse has a leg injury, the bedding must not be deep as it will drag on the limb when the horse moves around. In such cases, use minimal bedding on rubber matting if possible. However, if there is danger of the horse injuring himself further when lying down, a deep bed is essential.

The stable must be well ventilated to ensure a constant flow of fresh air and maintain the horse's respiratory health. Keep the top door open to allow fresh air in. Ideally, there should also be a window on the same side as the door, opening inwards, to encourage the air to lift upwards. A ventilation cowl in the roof allows warm, stale air to escape as it is replaced by cool fresh air. The stable must, however, be free of draughts or the horse will feel cold and may catch a chill. Draughts occur from gaps, particularly under the stable door and from odd holes in the walls.

In most conditions it is desirable for the stable to be naturally light. However, it may be necessary to keep a horse suffering from an eye injury or periodic opthalmia in a darkened stable.

The stable must be peaceful to allow the horse to rest quietly. Keep noise and activity around the sick horse's stable to a minimum.

ITQ 133 Describe how you will bed the stable for:

a. A horse on box rest after colic surgery.

b. A horse on box rest with a lower limb injury.

WARMTH

In cold weather the horse must be kept warm through the use of additional clothing rather than by closing the top door and window of the stable. Well-fitting rugs must be used as needed. Use layers of lightweight sheets rather than one heavy rug. This way you can adjust them easily. If the horse is prone to breaking out in a sweat, place a sweat/cooler sheet beneath his stable rug to help the air to circulate; alternatively a thermal rug can be used.

In very cold conditions a neck hood may be added.

Stable bandages applied over Gamgee also help to keep a horse warm.

These should be removed every 12 hours (or as specified by the vet if the legs are bandaged for support) and the legs hand-massaged to promote circulation.

In extremely cold weather, or when a horse is very sick, heat lamps/panels may be used. These are suspended above the horse, e.g. from a beam. Great care must be taken, particularly with heat lamps, as there is a fire risk. All wires must be safely out of the horse's reach and a circuit breaker plug used.

To check a horse for warmth, look for the following signs:

- Body heat – put your hand underneath the horse's rug to feel how warm he is. The horse should feel comfortably warm; not hot and damp with sweat. Lift the rug(s) and check his flanks to see if he is sweating.

- Ears should feel dry and warm, not cold or damp. If they feel very cold, use a towel and rub and pull the ears gently to help the circulation.

- The coat will be dull and staring if the horse is cold.

- Shivering – if very cold, the horse will shiver and look tucked-up and miserable.

> ITQ 134 List four points relevant to keeping the horse warm.
>
> 1.
>
> 2.
>
> 3.
>
> 4.

FEEDING

The sick horse must go immediately onto a non-heating diet, i.e. one low in carbohydrate and protein. If he is confined to the stable and still fed his normal working diet many problems could occur. These problems include:
- Exertional rhabdomyolysis (azoturia).
- Lymphangitis.
- Laminitis.
- Weight gain and inappropriate behaviour.

Good quality meadow hay is easily digested; this will keep the horse occupied and will not 'hot him up'. If the hay is put in a net with small holes it will take longer for the horse to pull the hay through these, so helping to occupy him. However, there are disadvantages to using haynets; the horse is eating in an unnatural position as the incisors do not align with each other when the head is raised. Also, having the head low, as when eating from the ground, encourages the clearance of bacteria and fluid from the lungs. This clearance is greatly reduced if the horse has his head raised for long periods. Grazing in hand is also beneficial to the horse for this reason, as well as providing a good source of forage.

If the horse has a dust allergy, shake all hay and soak for 10 minutes before feeding. If feeding a haylage product, choose a high-fibre, non-heating type.

Warm bran mashes are non-heating, palatable to an 'off-colour' horse and are easily digested. Add limestone flour to boost calcium levels. If a laxative effect is needed, add a tablespoon of Epsom salts. However, not all horses like the taste of Epsom salts. Alternatively, soak non-heating cubes in hot water to make a nutritionally balanced mash. Feed manufacturers produce compound feeds specifically for the recuperating horse so it is easy to feed a balanced and safe diet.

If a horse is not keen to eat, try offering a tasty treat such as sliced apples or carrots. Some horses enjoy molasses and freshly cut (not mown) grass.

If food is not eaten, remove it from the stable. Never leave uneaten food in the food bowl as it soon turns rancid and attracts flies and vermin. Offer very small quantities of food – horses can often be tempted by hand-feeding.

If the horse is eating well he can (if appropriate to his condition) be kept occupied by being fed using a feedball, a device which the horse has to move around to release small quantities of food.

A vitamin and mineral supplement may be needed as the horse will be consuming below his normal recommended daily amounts.

WATER

Use water buckets for the sick horse so that you can monitor the amount drunk. Switch off any automatic water supply in the stable but do make sure the horse has seen and will use the water buckets. If the horse refuses to use the buckets but will use the automatic drinker then obviously you will have to stick with the drinker.

Ensure that there is a constant supply of clean, fresh 'chilled' water. 'Chilled' water has, in fact, had a drop of hot water added to take the chill off. A drink of icy cold water could make a sick horse feel uncomfortable, possibly leading to abdominal pain.

Change the water frequently, especially if the horse has a nasal discharge that will taint it.

Add a small amount of glucose to the drinking water to give the horse an instant source of energy and nourishment. If the horse has been sweating profusely, or actually dehydrated, electrolytes can be added to the feed or water. If using electrolytes in the water, always have one bucket of plain water available to the horse so he can choose between them. Horses have to get used to the taste of electrolytes and not every horse will drink water with them added. If this is the case, and electrolytes have to be administered, this can be done via an oral syringe.

GROOMING

Pick out the feet twice daily to prevent thrush.

Whether or not you brush the horse over each day depends upon how sick he is. Generally, keep grooming to a minimum – however, a quick brush over with the body brush is good for circulation and hygiene. Check rugs for slipping and chafing. Massage the legs to improve circulation.

Wipe the eyes, nostrils and dock with separate clean, damp sponges. Each horse should have his own sponges and these must be regularly boiled in a disinfectant solution to kill bacteria.

If the ailment is contagious, such as strangles, wipe the eyes and nostrils with Gamgee swabs and dispose of the swabs after use.

Wash your hands before and after handling a sick horse.

BOREDOM

Boredom is a factor to consider with horses on box rest. To reduce boredom:

- Graze in hand several times a day if appropriate and safe to do so.
- Feed cut (not mown) grass and if possible, cut herbs such as comfrey.
- Feed several small feeds during the day.
- Taking into account the caveats previously mentioned, it may be helpful to use a haynet with small holes and a feedball.
- Install a stable mirror so that the horse can see his own reflection. Studies have proved that this helps reduce confinement stress.
- Spend time with the horse grooming and massaging him.
- Physiotherapy can begin in the stable.
- So long as the horse on box rest does not have a condition requiring isolation, stable a quiet horse in the box next door to allow the rested horse to communicate with another.

KEEPING VETERINARY RECORDS

A written record should be kept of vaccinations, worming, shoeing and general health. If a horse becomes sick, a daily record of the following should be kept:

- Visits by the vet, including diagnosis and treatment.
- The horse's condition, including clinical signs, temperature, pulse and respiratory rates.
- Treatments administered by you.
- Food and water intake.
- Whether droppings and urine are normal.

Always be observant, note any changes which occur so that you can give the vet all relevant information.

Insurance

Depending on the nature of the disease or injury, the owner of the horse may have to inform the insurance company as soon as the horse becomes sick or injured. It is important to read the policy in depth as failure to disclose information can invalidate certain types of insurance claim.

ADMINISTERING MEDICATION

Looking after a sick horse involves administering medication. The vet will always advise on the administration of medicines including:

- The type of drug.
- The correct dose.
- The method of administration.
- The frequency of administration.
- Duration of treatment.

However, in many cases it will be necessary or expedient for the horse's owner or yard staff to administer medication, so we will now look at the various ways in which this can be done.

Storing Medication

Drugs, treatments and dressings should be:

- Stored in a dust-proof container, such as a plastic storage box within a locked cupboard.
- Kept cool, dry and in a dark place. Drugs should not be exposed to bright sunlight or extremes of temperature.
- Kept out of the reach of children and unauthorized persons.
- Discarded when they reach their use-by dates. (When disposing of medication, check with the vet as to the safest method for each type of drug.)

METHODS OF ADMINISTRATION

The method by which medication is administered will mainly depend on the condition being treated and the type of drug. Routes of administration can be broadly divided into:

1. **Topical**: has a local effect and is administered directly where the action is required.
2. **Enteral:** the desired effect is systemic (not local) and the drug is given via the digestive tract.
3. **Parenteral:** the desired effect is systemic but the drug is administered via routes other than the digestive tract.

Topical Application

Epicutaneous application is application onto the skin. Examples include anti-bacterial creams, anti-inflammatory creams and cytotoxic creams (for sarcoid treatment).

Eye drops and creams, e.g. antibiotics used in the treatment of conjunctivitis.

Inhalation and nebulization. Inhalations are given to horses suffering from ailments of the respiratory tract to help clear any mucus and discharge from the airways. A decongestant such as Friar's balsam or eucalyptus oil is poured onto a small amount of hay in the bottom of a bucket. The bucket is placed into the bottom of a large hessian sack and boiling water is poured onto the hay. The horse is then encouraged to stand with his head in the sack so that he breathes in the vapours. More boiling water is poured onto the hay to produce more vapour. Whilst carrying out this procedure, make sure that the horse cannot touch the hot kettle.

A nebulizer converts the drug being administered into a vapour which the horse inhales through a specially designed mask. Drugs to be administered this way include sodium chromoglycate, which acts on the cells of the airways to reduce an allergic reaction.

Intravaginal or intrauterine administration. Certain conditions affecting the reproductive organs require the administration of fluids, often with antibiotics added, into the vagina or uterus. The area around the vulva and anus (the perineum) is washed and a catheter inserted either into the vagina or uterus. The fluid, which must be slightly below body temperature and sterile, is then poured or pumped in.

Pessaries are tablets containing antibiotics that are inserted into the vagina or uterus.

On the tongue. Some medicines, such as cough electuaries, can be put onto a wooden spatula. (A wooden spoon with the sides sawn off can be used). Open the horse's mouth and hold your fingers in one corner of the mouth to keep it open. Smear the electuary at the back of the tongue. This is not a commonly used method of administration.

Enteral Administration

Orally in the feed. Powders and liquids can be mixed in with dampened feed. Try to give the horse his favourite foods to tempt him and always give them to him at the normal times so as not to arouse his suspicions. Offer molasses, sliced apples or carrots to disguise the taste. If a horse has lost his appetite another method must be used.

Orally in paste form. Rather like the paste wormers, medicine can be squirted onto the back of the tongue by means of a plastic syringe. This method is ideal for a horse who is not eating or drinking very well and it ensures no wastage.

Orally in the water. Powders may be put into the water buckets provided the horse is drinking. This method cannot be used with automatic drinking bowls as you cannot tell if the horse has had a drink or not and medication may be wasted.

Intubation (nasogastric/stomach tube). The vet may decide to intubate when a horse is suffering from certain types of colic. Liquid paraffin may be administered to lubricate the contents of the digestive tract to ease an impaction. A length of rubber or plastic tube is passed up the nostril, through the pharynx and into the oesophagus. Swallowing helps to allow the tube into the oesophagus. If the tube is placed incorrectly into the trachea the fluid and/or drugs will be administered directly into the lungs, resulting in severe pneumonia or drowning. Because of this risk, this procedure is only carried out by the vet.

Enema. In conditions for which a large quantity of fluid needs to be administered, e.g. to aid evacuation of the rectum or colon, or in the treatment or prevention of dehydration, this method is useful.

The vet will first remove faeces from the rectum using a well-lubricated gloved hand. The tube used for administering the enema should be lubricated and is inserted into the rectum and gently passed forward. Warm fluid is slowly pumped into the rectum.

This method is sometimes used in foals suffering from meconium retention. A soft, narrow tube is used to administer warm, soapy water, paraffin or a commercially prepared solution to lubricate the meconium and aid its evacuation.

> **ITQ 135**
>
> a. What is intubation?
>
> b. Why is this procedure only to be carried out by a vet?

Parenteral Administration

Injections provide an effective method of getting the drug directly into the horse's system, so helping it to take effect more quickly. Injections are usually into either muscle (intramuscular) or into a vein (intravenous). In the treatment of certain conditions, injections may be given into a joint (intra-articular). Injections are normally given by the vet but, if a course of treatment is needed, an experienced person may, with the vet's permission, give intramuscular injections. (*Always seek the advice of the vet for instructions and guidance regarding intramuscular injections*).

INTRAMUSCULAR INJECTION

The intramuscular route is a simple and effective method of administering medication.

- Make sure the horse's coat is clean and dry. To inject through a dirty coat could introduce bacteria into the muscle and cause infection.
- Have an assistant to hold and restrain the horse. Have additional restraint equipment to hand, e.g. a twitch.
- Wash your hands.
- Read the instructions on the bottle and check the contents. Give the bottle a good shake.

- Wipe the rubber stopper of the bottle with cotton wool soaked in methylated or surgical spirit to clean it and remove bacteria.
- It is important that the needle and syringe are sterile. Keep the needle in its cover and attach it to the syringe.
- Remove the needle cover and make sure it doesn't touch anything else. If it does accidentally touch anything it must be discarded and another needle used.
- Hold the bottle upside down and push the needle through the stopper. The point of the needle should be immersed in the fluid.
- Withdraw the plunger and draw in more than is needed for the treatment. Still keeping the bottle upright, return the excess to the bottle. This gets rid of air from the syringe.
- Draw the needle out of the bottle and replace the needle cover.
- Wash any spillage from your hands immediately.

The muscles of the neck provide a good site for injecting so are most commonly used (see Figure 37). Measure one hand's breadth from the base of the neck and one hand's length from the line of the crest.

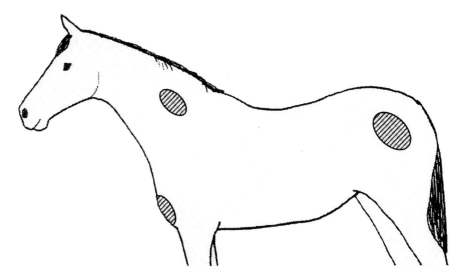

Figure 37 Sites for intramuscular injection

Table 4 (page 180) compares the merits of different sites for intramuscular injections.

Intramuscular injection method 1

1. The site may be swabbed with surgical or methylated spirit to help clean the area.
2. Remove the needle from the syringe and hold it between the thumb and first two fingers. Remove the needle cover.
3. Tap the horse a few times with the back of the hand near the injection site and with a positive action, insert the needle horizontally to its full depth.
4. There must be no bleeding from the site. If any blood appears it means the needle has inadvertently been placed into a blood vessel. The needle must be replaced and repositioned before giving the injection.

5. Attach the loaded syringe and pull the plunger back to check for blood. If blood is aspirated the needle should be replaced and repositioned.
6. If no blood is aspirated the injection may be given. Depress the plunger firmly, holding the needle and syringe together with the other hand to prevent them from being forced apart. You may need to exert considerable pressure on the plunger, especially if the suspension is quite thick.
7. Withdraw the needle. A small droplet of blood may appear – this is nothing to worry about.

Intramuscular injection method 2
1. The needle and syringe are left attached and the needle cover is removed.
2. Take a fold of skin in one hand and gently but positively insert the needle through the skin, deep into the muscle.
3. Pull the plunger back to check for blood and proceed as in method 1.

Method 2 is useful for horses who react badly to the insertion of the needle, e.g. fractious horses. The administration of intramuscular injections can, in fact, present certain problems. These, with guidelines to help resolve them, are:

- **Fractious horse**. Restrain the horse more positively, e.g. with a twitch. If the horse continues to throw himself around, leave him and consult the vet.

- **Aspiration of blood**. Certain drugs, e.g. some antibiotics, can be fatal if injected directly into the bloodstream. As previously explained, the needle should be repositioned before giving the injection.

- **Excess air in the syringe**. The top of the needle may not be immersed in the suspension, causing air from the bottle to be drawn in. Air can also enter the syringe where the needle and syringe are connected. *The air must be expelled from the syringe before inserting the needle.*

- **Broken needle**. If the needle breaks, take hold of the protruding part and withdraw it firmly. If you cannot remove it, mark the area and consult the vet.

- **Neck stiffness and soreness following injection**. The vet may need to prescribe phenylbutazone to relieve the inflammation. Food and water containers should be raised to make it easier for the horse to reach. To help reduce the incidence of neck soreness, use alternate sides of the neck if the treatment runs over several days.

- **Abscess formation**. This may occur as a result of contamination. The vet should be consulted.

SITE	ADVANTAGES	DISADVANTAGES
Neck	Ease of administration Thin skin – minimal force required Restraint is easier	May lead to neck stiffness Small muscle mass so not suitable for large dosage Proximity of nuchal ligament and cervical vertebrae
Gluteal	Large muscle mass – suitable for high-volume doses	Thicker skin – greater force required to inject Poor drainage if an abscess forms Administration more difficult in larger/fractious horses
Biceps femoris	Large muscle mass in foals	Except in the case of a foal, administration is difficult
Semi-membranosus/semi-tendinosus	Large muscle mass in foals Reasonable drainage if an abscess forms	Can be difficult to administer Sciatic nerve is in the region
Pectorals	Good drainage if an abscess forms Easy to administer small volumes	Tends to abscess more readily

Table 4 Comparisons of sites for intramuscular injection

ITQ 136 State the precautions necessary to prevent infection when administering an intramuscular injection.

ITQ 137

a. Describe how to check that the needle has not entered a blood vessel when giving an intramuscular injection.

b. Why is it essential to check this?

c. What will you do if blood appears at the needle hub or in the syringe?

ITQ 138 State two disadvantages of using the neck as a site for intramuscular injection.

1.
2.

INTRAVENOUS AND INTRA-ARTICULAR INJECTIONS

These injections are always given by the vet; intravenous injections are normally into one of the jugular veins. The needle, bottle and its contents must be sterile. The drug will take effect very quickly as it enters the circulatory system immediately.

RECOVERY AND REHABILITATION

After injury or illness there will be the need for a period of recovery and rehabilitation, the duration and nature of which will depend upon the severity of the condition. Post-operative recovery is a specialist subject requiring the expertise of the veterinary team and the clinic's facilities.

The main objectives of rehabilitation are:

- To restore to normality the injured tissue through repair and re-education (encouraging the restored tissue and attendant structures to function correctly).
- To improve strength and flexibility.
- To restore the normal range of movement.
- To increase athleticism and stamina.

Traditionally, the majority of horses were turned away to rest immediately after injury has occurred. However, if the injury was causing discomfort the horse would move in an unbalanced way to compensate. Such movement might well become established, leading to uneven muscular development and the development of an uneven gait, which would probably be maintained upon full recovery.

Also, under such a regime, as the horse is constantly moving out of balance the old injury is likely to recur or indeed, a new injury may result. Therefore, if it is possible to rehabilitate the horse before he is turned away to rest, his chances of a full and balanced recovery are greater and this should result in prolonged soundness. This rehabilitation process may be aided by physiotherapy.

PHYSIOTHERAPY

Physiotherapy is the science and application of anatomy, exercise physiology, histology, biomechanics, physics and psychology of a person or animal with an injury, pain, or dysfunction. Physiotherapy involves the assessment, treatment and rehabilitation of the patient, with the aim of return to full function and performance. This is achieved by utilizing manual therapies, electrotherapies and individual exercise and rehabilitation programmes.

During treatment and rehabilitation the physiotherapist, vet and owner will need to work together. In consultation with the vet, and with reference to the individual horse's condition, a physiotherapist will recommend suitable treatment options, some of which have been described in Chapter 3. The vet, physiotherapist and owner will then monitor the horse's reaction to treatment, and his progress. When the vet and physiotherapist are in agreement, re-education (the process towards bringing the horse back into work) can begin.

INTRODUCING EXERCISE

Whatever the method(s) used, all exercise must be built up gradually.

- **Walking in hand** ensures that the horse moves in a controlled manner, thereby reducing the risk of worsening the injury. Use a Chifney for extra control if the horse is lively. Walk on even surfaces, avoiding very tight turns and small circles. The horse must wear brushing boots all round and the handler should wear gloves, protective footwear and a crash cap. Consult the vet if the horse is likely to be very 'full of himself' as it may be necessary and desirable to sedate him. This improves handler safety and helps prevent the horse from re-injuring himself through wild behaviour.

- **Turn out** initially in a small cage or pen to prevent the horse moving around too much or building up speed. It may be beneficial to sedate the horse for the first few times he is turned out.

- **Horse-walker**. Walking can be introduced in the horse-walker. This is often safer as no handler is involved but, as with walking in hand, it is important the horse does not thrash about, as he could injure himself. On the horse-walker the horses are working on a constant circle which in some lameness rehabilitation programmes could be a disadvantage, as uneven pressure is exerted on the horse's muscles and limbs. Horses should work evenly on both reins on the walker.

- **Swimming** may be included in the rehabilitation programme. It is a useful form of exercise as the horse's limbs bear no weight. However, care must be taken to ensure that each limb is used evenly to promote even muscular development. As the limbs are not weightbearing, swimming does not develop the strength of tendons, ligaments or bone. A suitable heart rate monitor should be used as the horse may easily become stressed if unused to swimming. It should be noted that if it's the horse's first time in the pool his heart rate will be very high. Walking in water, particularly against a current, is also very beneficial. The sea is ideal, otherwise a safe stream or wading area at a pool can be used.

- **Long-reining** on straight lines at walk can, if carried out properly, help to even out muscular imbalances. In the early stages of a rehabilitation programme, excessive circle work would exert too much strain on the muscles, tendons, ligaments and joints.

- **Basic ridden schooling**, once a high level of recovery has been achieved, can supple and strengthen muscles as well as helping to improve balance. Steady work over raised poles improves rhythm and tempo whilst encouraging the horse to flex his joints effectively. At the riding stage of the rehabilitation programme, it is important to appreciate that correct shoeing, bitting, care of teeth and saddle fitting all affect the horse's chances of staying in balance.

- **Lungeing** should be carried out on an even, non-slip surface. Prior to lungeing the horse should be warmed up by walking in hand. The size of circle will depend on the horse's size and athletic ability, i.e. the larger/less athletic the horse, the larger the circle should be. A large circle is less demanding than a small circle so is appropriate at the start of the rehabilitation programme for all horses. If necessary, the person lungeing can themselves move, to prevent the horse working on too small a circle.

    Establish and maintain an even rhythm, working towards a relaxed, loose movement with the horse tracking up evenly on both reins. Variations within the gaits (i.e. some lengthening and shortening within the gaits) can be helpful.

    Never lunge for too long – start with short sessions, i.e. no more than 10 minutes initially and change the rein frequently.

    Preferably after reintroducing them on straight lines, trotting poles can be introduced on the lunge, starting with three poles flat on the ground, building up to several poles with one or both ends raised on blocks.

    Provided the handler is competent in their fitting and use, training aids such as the Pessoa training system and the Chambon can be useful when trying to encourage the horse to work correctly, thereby developing muscles evenly.

FURTHER CHECKS

Once the horse has recovered from the injury or illness, steps must be taken to maintain soundness and fitness.

- As the horse's exercise levels increase, his diet will need to be adjusted.

- The farrier will need to shoe to ensure optimum foot balance. The farrier may need to consult the vet when shoeing following limb/soundness problems.

- As the horse starts to build up muscle, saddle fit should be checked.

- The horse's teeth should be checked by an equine dentist or the vet.

Key points to consider with any horse as he recovers are to follow the vet's advice and treat each horse as an individual.

CHAPTER SUMMARY

Disease control is a significant aspect of yard management, but becomes even more important in large yards, particularly where there is regular movement of horses on and off the premises. This chapter described the main principles of disease control and isolation procedure.

The good horsemaster will recognize deviation from normal, thereby spotting problems promptly. Early recognition and appropriate liaison with the veterinary surgeon will improve the prognosis for all horses, whatever the problem.

Subsequent management of the sick horse will be influenced by the nature of the horse's disease or injury. The yard manager and horse's owner must work with the vet and, if appropriate, other healthcare professionals and the farrier, caring for the horse in accordance with their instructions.